Feeding Children Inside and Outside the Home

This cross-disciplinary volume brings together diverse perspectives on feeding children inside and outside of the home across different geographical locations. By unpacking mundane food occasions – from school dinners to domestic meals and from breakfast to snacks – *Feeding Children Inside and Outside the Home* shows the role of food in the everyday lives of children and adults around them. Investigating food occasions at home, schools and in nurseries during weekdays and holidays, this book reveals how children, mothers, fathers, teachers and other adults involved in feeding children, understand, make sense of and navigate ideological discourses of parenting, health imperatives and policy interventions.

Revealing the material and symbolic complexity of feeding children, and the role that parenting and healthy discourses play in shaping, perpetuating and transforming both feeding and eating, this volume shows how micro and macro aspects are at play in mundane and everyday practices of family life and education. This volume will be of great interest to a wide range of students and researchers interested in the sociology of family life, education, food studies and everyday consumption.

Vicki Harman is a Senior Lecturer in Sociology at the University of Surrey. Her research interests include family life in contemporary Britain and social divisions including gender, social class and ethnicity. Vicki has conducted qualitative research into food practices within families, focusing on feeding the family on a low or reduced income and parents' perspectives on preparing lunchboxes for their children. She has published her research in journals including *Sociology, Ethnic and Racial Studies, Identities: Global Studies in Culture and Power, Young Consumers, International Journal of Consumer Studies* and *The British Journal of Social Work*.

Benedetta Cappellini is a Senior Lecturer in Marketing and Consumer Behaviour at Royal Holloway, University of London. Her research interests are in food consumption, material culture, family consumption and motherhood and consumption. She has published in journals including *Sociology, The Sociological Review, Consumption, Markets and Culture, Journal of Marketing Management, Journal of Business Research,* and *Journal of Consumer Behaviour and Advances in Consumer Research*. She is the co-editor of *The Practice of the Meal: Families, food and the market place* (Routledge, 2016).

Charlotte Faircloth is a Lecturer in the Sociology of Gender at University College London. Her research interests include parenthood, infant feeding, gender, intimacy and equality. She has published in journals including *Sociology, The Sociological Review, Health, Risk and Society* and *Ethnos*. She is the author of *Militant Lactivism? Attachment parenting and intensive motherhood in the UK and France* (Berghahn Books, 2013), co-author of *Parenting Culture Studies* (Palgrave, 2014) and co-editor of *Parenting in Global Perspective: Negotiating ideologies of kinship, self and politics* (Routledge, 2013).

Sociological Futures

Sociological Futures aims to be a flagship series for new and innovative theories, methods and approaches to sociological issues and debates and 'the social' in the 21st century. This series of monographs and edited collections was inspired by the vibrant wealth of British Sociological Association (BSA) symposia on a wide variety of sociological themes. Edited by a team of experienced sociological researchers, and supported by the BSA, it covers a wide range of topics related to sociology and sociological research and will feature contemporary work that is theoretically and methodologically innovative, has local or global reach, as well as work that engages or reengages with classic debates in sociology bringing new perspectives to important and relevant topics.

The BSA is the professional association for sociologists and sociological research in the United Kingdom, with an extensive network of members, study groups and forums, and A dynamic programme of events. The Association engages with topics ranging from auto/biography to youth, climate change to violence against women, alcohol to sport, and Bourdieu to Weber. This book series represents the finest fruits of sociological enquiry, for a global audience, and offers a publication outlet for sociologists at all career and publishing stages, from well-established to emerging sociologists, BSA or non-BSA members, from all parts of the world.

Series Editors: Eileen Green, John Horne, Caroline Oliver, Louise Ryan

Social Mobility for the 21st Century
Everyone a winner?
Edited by Steph Lawler and Geoff Payne

Feeding Children Inside and Outside the Home

Critical Perspectives

Edited by
Vicki Harman, Benedetta Cappellini and Charlotte Faircloth

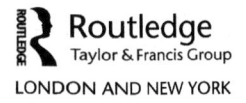

Routledge
Taylor & Francis Group
LONDON AND NEW YORK

First published 2019
by Routledge
2 Park Square, Milton Park, Abingdon, Oxon OX14 4RN

and by Routledge
711 Third Avenue, New York, NY 10017

Routledge is an imprint of the Taylor & Francis Group, an informa business

© 2019 selection and editorial matter, Vicki Harman, Benedetta Cappellini and Charlotte Faircloth individual chapters, the contributors

The right of Vicki Harman, Benedetta Cappellini and Charlotte Faircloth to be identified as the authors of the editorial material, and of the authors for their individual chapters, has been asserted in accordance with sections 77 and 78 of the Copyright, Designs and Patents Act 1988.

All rights reserved. No part of this book may be reprinted or reproduced or utilised in any form or by any electronic, mechanical, or other means, now known or hereafter invented, including photocopying and recording, or in any information storage or retrieval system, without permission in writing from the publishers.

Trademark notice: Product or corporate names may be trademarks or registered trademarks, and are used only for identification and explanation without intent to infringe.

British Library Cataloguing in Publication Data
A catalogue record for this book is available from the British Library

Library of Congress Cataloging in Publication Data
Names: Harman, Vicki, editor. | Cappellini, Benedetta, editor. | Faircloth, Charlotte, editor.
Title: Feeding children inside and outside the
home : critical perspectives / edited by Vicki Harman, Benedetta Cappellini and Charlotte Faircloth.
Description: Abingdon, Oxon ; New York, NY : Routledge, 2019.
Identifiers: LCCN 2018025984| ISBN 9781138633865 (hardback) | ISBN 9781315206974 (ebook)
Subjects: LCSH: Children--Nutrition--Cross-cultural studies. | Children--Nutrition--Psychological aspects. | Food habits--Cross-cultural studies.
Classification: LCC HQ784.E3 .F44 2019 | DDC 613.2083--dc23LC record available at https://lccn.loc.gov/2018025984

ISBN: 978-1-138-63386-5 (hbk)
ISBN: 978-1-315-20697-4 (ebk)

Typeset in Goudy
by Taylor & Francis Books

Contents

List of illustrations vii
List of contributors viii
Acknowledgements xiv
Foreword xv

1 Introduction 1
  VICKI HARMAN, CHARLOTTE FAIRCLOTH AND BENEDETTA CAPPELLINI

PART I
School and childcare settings 9

2 Unsettling food encounters between families and early
  childhood educators 11
  DEBORAH ALBON

3 Intersectionality and migrant parents' perspectives on preparing
  lunchboxes for their children 28
  VICKI HARMAN AND BENEDETTA CAPPELLINI

4 School meal reform and feeding ordering in Portugal:
  Conventions and controversies 42
  MÓNICA TRUNINGER AND ROSA SOUSA

5 "Don't bring me any chickens with sad wings": Discipline,
  surveillance, and "communal work" in peri-urban childcare
  centres in Cochabamba, Bolivia 63
  CARA DONOVAN, ALDER KELEMAN SAXENA, CAROL CARPENTER AND
  DEBBIE HUMPHRIES

PART II
The home (and beyond) — 85

6 Holiday hunger: Feeding children during the school holidays — 87
   PAMELA GRAHAM, PAUL STRETESKY, MICHAEL LONG, EMILY MANN AND MARGARET ANNE DEFEYTER

7 "My mum feeds me, but really, I eat whatever I want!": A relational approach to feeding and eating — 107
   ZOFIA BONI

8 Feeding in context: Eating occasions as domestic socialized practice — 124
   DAVID MARSHALL

PART III
New Parenting Styles? — 141

9 When fathers feed their family: The emergence of new father roles in Denmark — 143
   MALENE GRAM AND ALICE GRØNHØJ

10 Swedish single fathers feeding the family — 156
   SUSANNA MOLANDER

11 Calibrating motherhood — 174
   KATE CAIRNS, JOSÉE JOHNSTON AND MERIN OLESCHUK

12 When intensive mothering becomes a necessity: Feeding children on the ketogenic diet — 191
   MICHELLE WEBSTER

13 Concluding remarks — 207
   BENEDETTA CAPPELLINI, CHARLOTTE FAIRCLOTH AND VICKI HARMAN

Index — 211

Illustrations

Figures

4.1	Food service in nursery school	56
4.2	Food service in nursery school	57
4.3	Children eating around the table	57
4.4	Children eating around the table	58
6.1	Distribution of holiday hunger clubs by childhood depravation in England and Wales in 2016	100
8.1	Family meals and identity practice	133

Tables

4.1	Moral orders and school meals controversies	46
5.1	Child Centres Overview	68
5.2	Data Collection	70
6.1	Five Questions That Measure Holiday Hunger	98
9.1	Overview of sample and assessment of participation	147
10.1	Participants' profile	161

Contributors

Deborah Albon is Senior Lecturer in Early Childhood Studies at the University of Roehampton. Her main research interests centre on food and eating practices in early childhood settings. In particular she is interested in babies and young children's playful participation in the 'life' of their settings (through the lens of 'food events') as well as issues pertaining to the 'civilising' of children's bodies.

Zofia Boni is a social scientist, Assistant Professor at the Anthropology Department at Adam Mickiewicz University in Poznan, Poland, and a post-doctoral research associate at the SOAS Food Studies Centre in London, UK. She co-convenes the EASA Food Network. Her research interests include studying social relations and the moral implications entangled with children and food. Zofia's new research project takes a critical look at the social dynamics of childhood obesity in Poland. She has published in Anthropology of Food and *Children's Geographies*.

Kate Cairns is Assistant Professor of Childhood Studies at Rutgers University, USA. Her research investigates dynamics of gender, culture and inequality, with particular focus on the construction of children and youth as the promise of collective futures. Kate is co-author (with Josée Johnston) of *Food and Femininity* (Bloomsbury, 2015), and has published articles in venues such as *Gender & Society, Theory and Society, Journal of Consumer Culture*, and *Antipode*.

Benedetta Cappellini is a Senior Lecturer in Marketing and Consumer Behaviour at Royal Holloway, University of London. Her research interests are in food consumption, material culture, family consumption and motherhood and consumption. She has published in journals including *Sociology, The Sociological Review, Consumption, Markets and Culture, Journal of Marketing Management, Journal of Business Research, Journal of Consumer Behaviour* and *Advances in Consumer Research*. She is the co-editor of *The Practice of the Meal: Families, food and the market place* (Routledge, 2016).

List of contributors ix

Carol Carpenter is a Senior Lecturer and Associate Research Scholar in Environmental Anthropology at the School of Forestry & Environmental Studies and Adjunct Lecturer in the Anthropology Department at Yale University. Her teaching and research interests focus on the history and theory of environmental anthropology, the anthropology of conservation and sustainable development, applications of economic anthropology to environmental issues, and gender in agrarian and ecological systems. She spent four years in Indonesia engaged in urban household and community-level research on ritual, and four years in Pakistan working as a development consultant on social forestry and women in development issues for USAID and the World Bank, among others.

Margaret Anne Defeyter is Faculty Associate Pro-Vice Chancellor of Knowledge Exchange at Northumbria University. Greta has been at Northumbria University since 2003. In addition to her university role, she is also Director of the Healthy Living Lab at Northumbria University. Her current research interests are in food poverty, holiday hunger and food insecurity. She has received funding from the ESRC, the British Academy, the Wellcome Trust, and the Big Lottery, and funding from local authorities and industry. In 2015, she published the first evaluation of holiday breakfast clubs and in 2016 published a paper based on the Meals & More programme. In 2015, she was made a Fellow from the British Psychological Society. More recently, she won a Food Heroes Award (Sustain, 2016) for her research and evaluations on school breakfast clubs and holiday hunger. In 2017, the Healthy Living Lab won the British Psychology Public Engagement Award (North East) for knowledge exchange.

Cara Donovan has a dual master's degree in Public Health and Environmental Science from the School of Public Health and the School of Forestry and Environmental Studies at Yale University (MPH & MESc 2018). Her primary interests are in improving human health and the environment through sustainable food systems. Her MESc research explored the barriers and facilitators to access and utilization of nutritious native and traditional crops in child and infant feeding in Cochabamba, Bolivia. She also completed her MPH thesis research of food insecurity among individuals seeking treatment for substance use disorders in New Haven, Connecticut. Prior to her studies at Yale, Cara worked in a nonprofit organization on programs to improve food access in low-income neighborhoods in New Haven.

Charlotte Faircloth is a Lecturer in the Sociology of Gender at University College London. Her research interests include parenthood, infant feeding, gender, intimacy and equality. She has published in journals including *Sociology, The Sociological Review, Health, Risk and Society* and *Ethnos*. She is the author of *Militant Lactivism? Attachment parenting and intensive motherhood in the UK and France* (Berghahn Books, 2013), co-author of

Parenting Culture Studies (Palgrave, 2014) and co-editor of *Parenting in Global Perspective: Negotiating ideologies of kinship, self and politics* (Routledge, 2013).

Pamela Graham is a Vice Chancellor's Research Fellow and Associate Director of the Healthy Living Lab currently working within the Department of Social Work, Education and Community Wellbeing at Northumbria University. Pam is particularly interested in child and adolescent development and family health and wellbeing and has conducted research predominantly investigating the impact of school and community food interventions on various outcomes for children and families. In 2015, she co-authored the first paper to report on an evaluation of holiday breakfast clubs and has since written further papers on the topic of school and community holiday clubs.

Malene Gram is Associate Dean (education) at the Faculty of Social Sciences, Aalborg University. Her research interests are in consumer culture with a special interest in issues related to childhood, perceptions of children and family in relation to consumption and intergenerational relationships. Recently she has studied family negotiations, particularly the role of children in family food purchase, student food consumption, and the consumption of family holidays. She has published in journals such as *Journal of Consumer Culture, Journal of Contemporary Ethnography, Journal of Youth Studies, Food, Culture and Society, International Journal of Consumer Studies, Advertising and Society Review*, and *Childhood*.

Alice Grønhøj is Associate Professor in Consumer Behaviour at Department of Management, School of Business and Social Sciences at Aarhus University. Her research interests include consumer socialisation, intergenerational transfer of consumer behaviour, family decision-making, and methodologies of marketing research related to pro-environmental consumption and healthy eating habits. She has received both national and EU grants on these topics and publishes in journals such as *Psychology & Marketing, Journal of Consumer Behaviour, Journal of Macromarketing*, and *Journal of Environmental Psychology*.

Ulla Gustafsson carried out research in the primary health care field before joining University of Roehampton, with a focus upon health promotion and work organisation. She has since conducted comparative analysis of public health policy in Sweden and the UK as well as studies into school meals. Ulla collaborated on a Food Standards Agency funded study evaluating methods for including 'hard-to-reach' populations in food policy developments and is the co-editor of a Special Issue on *Food for Critical Public Health*. Current research interests include the role of food in everyday practice.

Vicki Harman is a Senior Lecturer in Sociology at University of Surrey. Her research interests include family life in contemporary Britain and social divisions including gender, social class and ethnicity. Vicki has conducted qualitative research into food practices within families, focusing on feeding the family on a low or reduced income and parents' perspectives on preparing lunchboxes for their children. She has published her research in journals including *Sociology, Ethnic and Racial Studies, Identities: Global Studies in Culture and Power, Young Consumers, International Journal of Consumer Studies* and the *British Journal of Social Work*.

Debbie Humphries has a broad background in public health research and practice. She has been a consultant in the areas of diet and physical activity behavior change, sustainability of community health programs, program monitoring and evaluation, and training in participatory monitoring and evaluation for organizations in Vietnam, Africa and in the United States. Her research addresses public health nutrition issues, interactions between nutrition and infectious disease, and programmatic approaches to improving public health.

Josée Johnston is Professor of Sociology at the University of Toronto. Her major substantive interest is the sociological study of food, which is a lens for investigating questions relating to consumer culture, gender, and inequality. She is the co-author of *Foodies* (2nd edition, Routledge, 2015) with Shyon Baumann, and has published articles in venues including *American Journal of Sociology, Journal of Consumer Culture, Signs, Theory and Society*, and *Gender and Society*.

Alder Keleman Saxena is an environmental anthropologist whose research explores the relationships linking agricultural biodiversity to food culture and nutritional health in the Bolivian Andes. In her research, she uses a mixed-methods, biocultural approach, which combines ethnography, ethnobotany, and public health nutrition. Alder recently defended her dissertation in fulfillment of the requirements for the combined degree program between the Yale School of Forestry & Environmental Studies, the Yale Department of Anthropology, and the New York Botanical Garden. Prior to her PhD, Alder worked in applied agricultural development research, focusing on the impacts of policy, technology development, and economic change on the diversity of maize landraces in Mexico.

Michael Long is an Associate Professor in Sociology at Oklahoma State University. He is interested in research methods and statistics and researches issues related to food insecurity, fair trade and environmental sustainability. His recent books include *The Treadmill of Crime: Green crime and political economy* (with P. Stretesky and M. Lynch, Routledge, 2013).

Emily Mann is a Psychology PhD student at Northumbria University, whose programme of research explores holiday hunger and evaluates the impact of holiday provision clubs on children and their families. As part of her research she has mapped the location and types of holiday provision clubs in the UK.

David Marshall is a Professor of Marketing and Consumer Behaviour at the University of Edinburgh Business School. His primary research interests include research on food access and availability; consumer food choice and eating rituals; and children's discretionary consumption in relation to food advertising and marketing. He edited *Understanding Children as Consumers* (Sage, 2010) and *Food Choice and the Consumer* (Springer, 1995) and has published in a number of academic journals including *The Sociological Review, Journal of Marketing Management, Consumption, Markets and Culture, Journal of Consumer Behaviour, International Journal of Advertising and Marketing to Children (Young Consumers), Appetite, Food Quality and Preference, International Journal of Epidemiology,* and *Journal of Human Nutrition*.

Susanna Molander is an Assistant Professor at the Centre for Fashion Studies, Stockholm University. Her research focuses on consumer culture with a particular interest in theories of practice and issues related to food, motherhood, fatherhood and consumption. She also studies fashion branding from a cultural perspective. With the Nordic context as her primary empirical base, she explores how political projects shape the way consumption is enacted.

Merin Oleschuk is a PhD candidate in the Department of Sociology at the University of Toronto. Her interests involve how intersecting inequalities shape family food habits, and the ways that disparate methodological tools can be applied to understand them. Her dissertation examines the relationship between cooking values and practices and their implications for the health behaviours of families.

Paul Stretesky is a Professor in the Department of Social Sciences, Northumbria University, and a member of the Healthy Living Lab. He investigates issues related to environmental and social justice. He has co-authored the following recent books: *Green Criminology: Crime, justice and the environment* (with M. Lynch, M. Long, & K. Barrett, University of California Press, 2017) and *Defining Crime: A critique of the concept and its implications* (with M. Lynch and M. Long, Palgrave, 2015). His recent articles appear in *Ecological Economics; Society & Natural Resources; Globalizations;* and *Health & Social Care in the Community*.

Rosa Sousa is a PhD candidate at the Climate Change and Sustainable Development Policies at the ICS-ULisboa. Her PhD research is looking at sustainable public procurement and school meals policies and initiatives in Portugal.

Mónica Truninger is a sociologist and senior research fellow at the Instituto de Ciências Sociais da Universidade de Lisboa (ICS-ULisboa). Her research interests are on children and eating practices, school meals, sustainable consumption and food provisioning systems. Together with Margit Keller, Bente Halkier and Terhi-Anna Wilska she has co-edited the *Routledge Handbook on Consumption*, published in 2017 (Routledge).

Michelle Webster is a Lecturer in Sociology at Royal Holloway, University of London. Her doctoral research focused on the experience and management of childhood epilepsy in the family and she has published findings from this study in *Sociology of Health and Illness* and *Social Science and Medicine*. Michelle is particularly interested in the experience of using dietary treatments for chronic conditions and the role that food consumption and food practices play in forming and maintaining social relationships.

Acknowledgements

The authors wish to thank all of the presenters and participants at their event, 'Feeding children inside and outside the home: Critical perspectives' which was held in London in March 2016. We are also grateful to Royal Holloway, Roehampton University and the UCL Institute of Education for their support in hosting that event. Many thanks too to our reviewers and editors at Routledge and in the BSA publications team – we are delighted to be able to include this volume in the Sociological Futures series. We are grateful to the contributors for working with us on this project and for their stimulating and thought-provoking chapters.

Vicki Harman and Benedetta Cappellini wish to thank the many parents they have met over the years of doing various pieces of fieldwork on families and food. Without their generosity, their work on this subject would not be possible. We would also like to thank the British Academy (SG130891) and Royal Holloway for funding the research on which Chapter 3 is based.

Charlotte Faircloth specifically wishes to thank Vicki Harman and Benedetta Cappellini for leading on this project during the period of her maternity leave.

Each of us would also like to thank our friends, families and colleagues for their encouragement and support.

Foreword

Feeding children is a mundane everyday activity that is vital for survival both on an individual level and of that as a species. It is not surprising therefore that there has long been a keen interest in the nutritional content of children's diets to ensure a healthy population, not the least in school meals policies. However, eating is not just about the physiological and the material but reflects powerful symbolic social and cultural meanings. The anthropologist Audrey Richards is credited as the pioneer in linking nutrition with social organisation as early as the 1930s, although her work was overlooked until the late 20th century. It is in extending the focus beyond nutrition where Harman, Cappellini and Faircloth are able to bring to the fore the complex world of feeding children inside and outside of the home through the contributions to this volume.

Children and food have been the object of sociological study for some decades, but the bringing together of studies addressing children and eating inside as well as outside the home and across cultures provide us with a fresh perspective on pertinent issues. Food serves as a good lens through which to explore social relations and values and the editors have put together a sensitive collection of material that points to the pressures when feeding children outside the home, the links between eating inside and outside the home, and the moral judgements often imposed upon or felt by parents in the choice of food or manners of eating.

In the late 1990s and early 2000s, when I set out to study school meals policy in the UK, (see, for example, Gustafsson 2004) the rationale in policy discussions, and in much of its associated campaigning, centred on children being sufficiently nourished to benefit from the education provided. It soon became evident that other concerns were implicit, including the conceptualisation of children over time, the relationship between the state and the family as well as that between children and parents. Of particular note was the lack of consideration of the children's perspective on the delivery of school meals, where it was clear they felt the only potential space they had to themselves was highly regulated. The volume develops these and other themes providing insights into what are often perceived as routine and everyday activities.

In this collection school meals policy and delivery are discussed in several papers. In Portugal, Truninger and Sousa reveal the broader political context and its impact on school meals and how this relates to children living with food insecurity. The authors accentuate how children and school food is an area of compromise. The child centres in Bolivia that are set up in order to address malnutrition and support mothers with childcare highlight the surveillance employed over participants while also grappling with the moral meanings attached to food (Donovan et al.). The outcome suggests a failure in achieving the intended purposes. Graham et al. remind us of the risks for social exclusion integral to schemes set up to deal with hunger, in this instance hunger during school holidays. While 'access to all' reduces potential stigma, scarce resources may serve to limit access to those in most need. Public initiatives aimed at feeding children are therefore fraught with contradictions as well as moral and political judgements.

When considering the interaction between feeding children inside and outside the home broader social value systems are in evidence. Harman and Cappellini's work on children's lunchboxes make explicit the fusion between private and public feeding of children. Normative and class based values are revealed as is the persistence of gendered expectations on women as providers. Albon too demonstrates how family life and values are also revealed through children's eating practices in early childhood settings where they become exposed to judgements by professionals. Families that do not correspond to idealised patterns then risk being marginalised. It is evident that feeding children inside the home provides an important context forming a basis for children's understanding of eating practices. Marshall identifies how children develop a 'self' as well as become part of a 'collective' through relations around eating between adults and children in the UK, while Boni's Polish study adds the way children formulate their own practices and preferences. Combining evidence from studies exploring feeding children outside and inside the home offer novel insights into the way diverse norms are created and assessed.

Gender is one of the key themes in the collection where the majority of expectations around feeding children are placed on mothers. Cairns et al. demonstrate the difficulty women face when feeding their children as they have to avoid both 'junk' food and being overly health conscious to escape criticism. Webster's study of mothers as expert carers of children with epilepsy identifies a case where not engaging with intensive parenting is not an option. In the main, most of the above studies suggest women's role in feeding children is expected. The volume adds to our understanding of gender and feeding children by also including work on fathers' accounts. Indeed Gram's Danish example suggests we need to acknowledge the input of fathers as part of action to tackle gender inequalities in the contribution to the household. Molander's Swedish findings identify a more relaxed approach to feeding children based on fathers' interest in food rather than the imperative of looking after their children. Such insights are important in terms of developing sociological understandings in a changing world but also suggest that perhaps expectations of fathers is such that whenever they take on a 'female' associated task they are going to be judged in a more favourable light than women.

This book provides a critical exploration of norms, values and social practices associated with feeding children. It is an innovative addition to a growing sociological literature in the area by bringing together examples considering feeding children inside and outside the home. It does this in a variety of contexts as well as geographical settings, while reflecting on the surveillance, moralities and values associated with this mundane everyday social practice. This is a sociologically informed collection drawing on interdisciplinary approaches where links and interactions between macro and micro settings and agendas are revealed. The collection is a welcome consolidation and challenge to future theoretical inquiries into feeding children.

Ulla Gustafsson,
University of Roehampton

Reference

Gustafsson, U. (2004) The privatisation of risk in school meals policies. *Health, Risk & Society*, 6(1) 53–66.

Chapter 1

Introduction

Vicki Harman, Charlotte Faircloth and Benedetta Cappellini

The current sociological literature on food and family life highlights how feeding children is now well-established as an everyday activity suffused with moral discourses of 'good' and 'bad' parenting (see, for example, DeVault 1991; Moisio et al. 2004; Miller 2005; Cairns et al. 2013) Expert guidance and mechanisms of surveillance and self-surveillance have been reported as common aspects of parenting (Faircloth 2010; The VOICE Group 2010; Elliot and Hore 2016). We see the growing extension of this surveillance and self-surveillance as a new form of intensive parenting (expanded in both time and space) whose consequences for family life, gendered identities and childhood have not been fully investigated (Faircloth 2014; Harman and Cappellini 2015; Harman and Cappellini 2017). Furthermore, academic debates are often restrained within academic disciplines, and as such, a broader understanding of the complexities of feeding children is missing.

In looking beyond the nutritionist-driven approach which largely sees feeding children as simply a matter of providing 'healthy' food, this edited book aims to provide new critical approaches to feeding children as a social practice influenced by a variety of institutions, norms, values and moral accountability. In particular, this collection seeks to provide an interrogation of contemporary parenting culture across geographical contexts. As such, the book sets out to examine the everyday practices of feeding and eating inside and outside the home. This collection aims to contribute to the literature on feeding the family and feeding children by engaging with theoretical debates around the moralization of feeding and eating practices, intensive parenting and everyday food consumption practices. This provides a timely and interdisciplinary reflection on government and marketplace discourses of feeding children, as well as their relations to the micro and macro politics of family life. It also aims to understand how parents and children interpret and sometimes challenge messages from health campaigns, governments, peers and others, as well as demonstrating change and continuity over time within individual experiences. As such, the book contributes to the growing body of literature on the changing nature of parenting culture.

Changing parenting culture and changing childhoods

Parenting has long been considered of the utmost significance when it comes to passing on social norms and values and continuing kinship, family and community life (Barlow and Chapin 2010). Recent sociological work has situated 'parenting' as critical for understanding contemporary changes in modern society – particularly in the US and the UK but increasingly in other contexts also. (Faircloth, Hoffman and Layne 2013). Drawing attention to wider sociocultural processes that have positioned modern child rearing as a highly important yet problematic sphere of social life, it can be argued that raising children has become a more complex task than it used to be in the past. Far from simply ensuring the transition to adulthood, today's parents are expected to do much more to secure and maximise the educational, social and physical development of their children (Lee et al. 2014). There are continuities with the past here, in that parenting has always been subject to moralizing advice and 'guidance', but the volume of the increase in expectations around raising children, particularly since the mid-1970s, is striking: parenting classes, parenting manuals, parenting experts, and parenting 'interventions' are now so common-place as to be unremarkable (Lee et al. 2014).

Based on a deterministic model of infant development, itself dependent on the growth of developmental psychology in the mid twentieth century, there is an assumption that infant experience is formative and underpins success or failure in adult life. Parenting is invoked as the source of, and solution to, a whole range of problems – at both individual, and social levels (such as the 'obesity epidemic'). There is particular concern over 'damage' in this vulnerable period, and an increasing focus on what has been called early-intervention or 'neuro-parenting' (Macvarish 2016). Rather than being something that is simple, straightforward or common sense, parenting is routinely presented as a task requiring expert guidance and supervision, particularly for those in lower socio-economic groups. Child rearing has become increasingly mediated through a cultural narrative that provides parents with rules – albeit hard to achieve and sometimes contradictory ones – about how to fulfill their roles as mothers and fathers. It is these rules that constitute 'parenting culture' (Lee et al. 2014). Of course, advice and guidance might well be appreciated by parents, particularly as it relates to 'the basics' of childcare; here, however, we are interested in the implications of this expansion of 'parenting' into an expertise-saturated, policy-focused and commercially fueled area of social life, particularly as it relates to feeding children.

As Lee and Furedi (2005) point out, the choices parents make today as to how to feed their children are often understood within this wider arena of debates about health, showing how, in the past few decades, the promotion of 'healthy living' has received enormous attention. As Fitzpatrick argues, '"Health" has come to operate as a "secular moral framework" for society, emphasizing individual responsibility and ... compliance with the appropriate medically sanctioned standard of behaviour' (2004:70). Framed as an area where outcomes are the result of individual and family choices, structural inequalities and material and social conditions are downplayed within these debates (Petersen and Lupton 1996). Healthy lifestyles become an expression of engagement with a particular political regime and a form of self-expression for the responsible citizen (Petersen and Lupton 1996) and more acutely, the expression of a responsible parent.

Part of the new health paradigm is an injunction to the individual to minimise risks from so-called 'bad' foods. As children are positioned as innocent and vulnerable within such debates, this carries moral implications for parents. Given the gendered distribution of food work (DeVault 1991 Cairns and Johnston 2015) the effect is felt particularly heavily by mothers, and the moralisation of eating intersects with the social construction of motherhood (Lee 2007; see also Lupton 1996). This is despite the fact that dual working families are now the norm, raising questions about how families negotiate food work and paid employment (O'Connell and Brannen, 2016). In recognizing the gendered dimension to these shifts, much work has drawn on the concept of 'intensive mothering' (Hays 1996) in understanding the experiences of contemporary women, who are increasingly 'torn' between the spheres of work and home – as well as theorizing how and why certain everyday tasks of childrearing, such as feeding have become moralized sources of heated public debate (Faircloth 2013; Hays 1996; Lee et al. 2014). Whilst this is most clearly obvious in the case of *infant* feeding (including debates around the benefits of breastfeeding or formula feeding) such antagonism around children's eating in general is increasingly visible in discussions of 'healthy' versus 'junk' food in childhood.

Arguing that the mother–child relationship represents a sacred bastion in a society otherwise governed by the pursuit of profit, Hays summarizes the characteristics of intensive motherhood, as 'child-centred, expert-guided, emotionally absorbing, labour intensive, and financially expensive' (Hays 1996: 8). Fathers have not been immune from this trend towards a more 'intensive' style of parenting, but it remains mothers to whom these cultural messages are largely targeted, and around women's reproductive choices that the fiercest debates reign. The child-centered 'intensive' mother is one who is considered responsible for all aspects of her child's development – physical, social, emotional and cognitive – above and beyond anyone else, including the father (Hays 1996:46). Ideally she demonstrates this commitment through embodied means, such as by breastfeeding, and no cost, physical or otherwise, is considered too great in her efforts to optimize her child (Wolf 2011).

The literature on changing parenting culture draws on important traditions within sociology around not only the 'doing' and 'display' of family (Finch 2007) but also individualisation and risk-consciousness (Beck and Beck-Gernsheim 1995, 2002). Indeed, one of the main features of this model, chiming with work done by modernization theorists (Beck 1992;

Giddens 1999) is that although children are safer than ever (materially at least) they are seen to be particularly vulnerable to risk in the early years, and must be protected and catered to by their mother at all times, lest their development be compromised. In a 'neo-liberal' era, with its emphasis on self-management, 'good' mothers are reflexive, informed consumers, able to 'account' for their parenting strategies (Murphy 2003). Arguably, children have become not only 'lifestyle projects' but also a site of women's 'identity-work' (Faircloth 2013).

Being an 'involved' mother means more than merely being available, as it did for the 1950s housewife. Today, child rearing has become a full-time activity about which mothers are expected to be highly informed and reflexive. In a period of 'intensive' parenting, permeated by processes of individualization, parenting must continually be reflected upon and the individual is assigned responsibility for ensuring that his or her parenting is 'good enough'. Of course, the perception of what is a 'good parent' is largely culturally, historically and ideologically rooted, and thus subject to continuous change. So this cultural script does not affect all parents in the same way around the world – social class, ethnicity and gender all affect its internalization, and there may be a curious combination of adoption, resistance or adaptation according to specific time and place, as this cross-culturally informed collection so aptly demonstrates. What is important, nevertheless, is that this script is increasingly recognized by parents in many geographical contexts as the 'proper' way of parenting, an injunction to which they must respond (Arendell 2000). As fathers' roles in society change (see, for example, Dermott 2008), more information is needed about the extent to which they too are influenced by these processes in key areas such as feeding children.

Parenting, in most areas of everyday life, is now considered to have a determining impact on a child's future happiness, healthiness, and success, and we suggest that feeding serves as a case-study par-excellence by which to explore this trend. As historical studies indicate, how babies and children are fed has long been construed as a matter of public debate and public interest (Kukla 2005; Murphy 2003). Yet as the accounts of many parents featured within the research in this collection show, public surveillance and monitoring of maternal decisions has certainly not receded, regardless of drastic declines in infant mortality and morbidity associated with very early childhood in the past. This monitoring is stronger than ever and has become connected to an ever-widening set of claims about children's 'success' or 'failure'. Even the biological core of a person – their brain – has come to be viewed as profoundly and directly impacted by the way that person was fed as a baby (O'Connor and Joffe 2013). This collection therefore makes a timely contribution to thinking not only about parenting, but also our very notions of personhood and social reproduction.

Summary of the contributions

This edited book brings together a collection of chapters exploring feeding children inside and outside of the home across a range of socio-cultural and geographical contexts (from homes in Poland, Sweden, Denmark, England and Canada to schools and childcare settings in Portugal, England and Bolivia). Although sociologically informed, this is an inter-disciplinary conversation taking into account perspectives from sociological, anthropological, socio-historical and interpretive consumer research. Such a conversation seeks to address the following questions: *What pressures are experienced when feeding children outside the home? To what extent do they build on, converge with or differ from those experienced in the domestic sphere? What are the implications for parental subjectivity when childhood eating has become so moralised?*

The answers to these questions have been organised in three main sections. In Part 1, focusing on feeding children in schools and childcare settings, the authors provide new insights into the dynamics of feeding and eating practices outside of the home. In Chapter 2, Deborah Albon draws upon ethnographic research in two early childhood settings in order to draw out some of the key differences in food practices in these contexts. She shows how children's eating practices conjure up particular images of family life, with the same practice (for example, finishing off breakfast from home 'on the go') being seen very differently in each context. She points to the importance of taking into account social class and ethnicity (of both the families and the educators), power differentials and the type of setting. Her attention to social class and ethnicity shares some synergies with Chapter 3 where Vicki Harman and Benedetta Cappellini draw upon interviews with migrant parents preparing packed lunches for their children in order to highlight how the mundane practice of selecting food to be consumed at school reveals much about families intersectional social identities. Following this, in Chapter 4 Mónica Truninger and Rosa Sousa examine school meal reform in Portugal. They focus on two key areas: how school meals are organised and children's tastes. Their chapter highlights the importance of questions relating to how food is transported and served, as well as what children eat. This also draws our attention to some of the disputes and compromises evident in the process of feeding children in a school setting. In Chapter 5, Cara Donovan and colleagues explore the experiences of directors and food preparers at childcare centres in Bolivia. Their work shows how the scrupulous medical monitoring and surveillance of children's bodies operated by different actors at the centres imposes hard-to-achieve targets onto families, and especially mothers.

Part 2 of this volume, titled 'The home (and beyond)', focuses on domestic eating practices experienced by children and their families, but understands these as being connected to wider social structures and social processes. Providing a link between the section on the home and that concerning the school, in Chapter 6 Pamela Graham and colleagues explore the issue of food poverty and feeding children during the school holidays. They review existing health and science literature to examine the potential impact of holiday hunger on childhood wellbeing before examining the way communities and local governments have established 'holiday clubs' to try to ameliorate this problem. Important questions are asked about whether these clubs should be available to all or only those most in need. Next, in Chapter 7, Zofia Boni shares her ethnographic research on foodways in Warsaw and argues for a relational approach to feeding and eating. Her findings paint a rich picture of feeding and eating practices and the relationship between the two. Following this, in Chapter 8, David Marshall focuses on children's perspectives on family meals and eating as a domestic socialized practice. He argues that children generally appear to be embracing family meals as an important part of family practices. He suggests that there appears to be relatively little conflict in children's accounts although they reported increased input regarding specific parts of the family meal.

Part 3 of this volume, titled 'New parenting styles?', draws our attention to potential new practices, ideas, ideals and understandings visible through research on parenting and food. In Chapter 9, Malene Gram and Alice Grønhøj explore fathers' participation in food work based upon a qualitative study conducted in Denmark. They argue that focusing solely or mainly on mothers' accounts risks men's housework being seen as invisible or undervalued. Interviewed in a family setting, fathers featured in their chapter were found to be actively involved and responsible for food work in a number of areas. In Chapter 10, Susanna Molander also considers fathers' participation in food work by focusing on the perspectives of single fathers in Sweden. She found that overall, the fathers in her study had a rather laid back approach to cooking and it was their own cooking interest and capabilities that emerged as point of departure rather than their role as parents. She argues that perhaps this mode of relaxed fathering can lead the way to a kind of caring that is not judged so harshly, by the parents themselves or by society at large.

Picking up on the notion of judgement, in Chapter 11 Kate Cairns, Josée Johnston and Merin Oleschuk discuss two pathologized and polarized extremes with regard to food work: the image of the woman who feeds her children only 'junk food' and the overbearing 'Organic Mom'. They highlight the difficulty for mothers in walking a moral tightrope when trying to avoid stigmatization with regard to food work, with insecurity, frustration and guilt as often-present emotions. Following this, in Chapter 12 Michelle Webster focuses on parenting practices when implementing the ketogenic diet – a diet high in fat and low in carbohydrates used to treat epilepsy. This chapter explores how the diet is incorporated into family life and the gendered nature of this incorporation. Additionally, this chapter illuminates how mothers were expert carers; experts in implementing the diet, experts on their own children's food tastes and experts at treating their child's condition. One key point to emerge from this chapter is that intensive parenting is not always the result of cultural ideology, but it can be the result of particular situations such as treating epilepsy through the ketogenic diet. Finally, in Chapter 13 we bring together the overall themes emerging from the collection and make some suggestions for future research.

References

Arendell, T. (2000) 'Conceiving and investigating motherhood: The decade's scholarship'. *Journal of Marriage and the Family*, 62(4): 1192–1207.
Barlow, K. and Chapin, B.L. (2010) 'The practices of mothering: An introduction'. *Journal of the Society for Psychological Anthropology*, ETHOS 38(4): 324–338.
Beck, U. (1992) *Risk Society: Towards a New Modernity*. New Delhi: SAGE.
Beck, U. and Beck-Gernsheim, E. (1995) *The Normal Chaos of Love*. Oxford: Polity Press.
Beck, U. and Beck-Gernsheim, E. (2002) *Individualization*. London: SAGE.
Cairns, K., Johnston, J. and MacKendrick, N. (2013) 'Feeding the "organic child": Mothering through ethical consumption'. *Journal of Consumer Culture*, 13(2): 97–118.
Cairns, K., and Johnston, J. (2015) *Food and Femininity*. London, New York: Bloomsbury Academic.
Dermott, E. (2008) *Intimate Fatherhood*, London and New York: Routledge.
DeVault, M. (1991) *Feeding the Family: The Social Organisation of Caring as Gendered Work*. Chicago, IL: University of Chicago Press.
Elliott, V. and Hore, B. (2016) '"Right nutrition, right values": the construction of food, youth and morality in the UK government 2010–2014'. *Cambridge Journal of Education*, 46(2): 177–193.
Faircloth, C. (2010) 'What science says is best: Parenting practices, scientific authority and maternal identity'. *Sociological Research Online Special Section on 'Changing Parenting Culture'*, 15(4).
Faircloth, C. (2013) *Militant Lactivism? Attachment Parenting and Intensive Motherhood in the UK and France*. Oxford and New York: Berghahn Books.
Faircloth, C. (2014) 'Intensive parenting and the expansion of parenting' 25–51. In Lee, E.Bristow, J.Faircloth, C. and Macvarish, J. (eds.) *Parenting Culture Studies*. Basingstoke and New York: Palgrave Macmillan.
Faircloth, C., Hoffman, D. and Layne, L. (eds.) (2013) *Parenting in Global Perspective: Negotiating Ideologies of Kinship, Self and Politics*. London: Routledge.
Finch, J. (2007) 'Displaying families'. *Sociology*, 41(1): 165–181.
Fitzpatrick, M. (2004) *MMR and Autism: What Parents Need to Know*. London: Routledge.
Giddens, A. (1999) 'Risk and responsibility'. *Modern Law Review*, 62(1): 1–10.
Harman, V. and Cappellini, B. (2015) 'Mothers on display: lunchboxes, social class and moral accountability'. *Sociology*, 49(4): 764–781.
Harman, V. and Cappellini, B. (2017) 'Boxed up? Lunchboxes and expansive mothering outside home'. *Families, Relationships and Societies*. www.ingentaconnect.com/content/tpp/frs/pre-prints/content-ppfrsd1600035r3 Advanced access published online 14. 08. 17.
Hays, S. (1996) *The Cultural Contradictions of Motherhood*. New Haven, CT: Yale University Press.

Kukla, R. (2005) *Mass Hysteria: Medicine, Culture and Women's Bodies*. New York: Rowman & Littlefield.

Lee, E. (2007). 'Infant Feeding in Risk Society', *Health, Risk and Society* 9(3), 295–309.

Lee, E.Bristow, J.Faircloth, C. and Macvarish, J. (2014) *Parenting Culture Studies*, Basingstoke and New York: Palgrave Macmillan.

Lee, E. and Furedi, F. (2005) '"Mothers" Experience of, and Attitudes to, Using Infant Formula in the Early Months'. School of Sociology, Sociology and Social Research: University of Kent at Canterbury. Retrieved 4 September 2006 from http://www.kent.ac.uk/sspssr/staff/academic/lee/infantformula-summary.pdf

Lupton, D. (1996) *Food, the Body and the Self*. London: Sage.

Macvarish, J. (2016) *Neuroparenting: The Expert Invasion of Family Life*. Basingstoke: Palgrave Macmillan.

Miller, T. (2005) *Making Sense of Motherhood: A Narrative Approach*. Cambridge: Cambridge University Press.

Moisio, R.Arnould, E. and Price, L. (2004) 'Between mothers and markets: constructing family identity through homemade food'. *Journal of Consumer Culture*, 4 (3): 361–384.

Murphy, E. (2003) 'Expertise and forms of knowledge in the government of families'. *Sociological Review*, 51(4): 433–462.

O'Connor, C. and Joffe, H. (2013) 'Media representations of early human development: Protecting, feeding and loving the brain'. *Social Science and Medicine*, 97: 297–306.

O'Connell, R. and Brannen, J. (2016) *Food, Families and Work*. London: Bloomsbury Academic.

Petersen, A. and Lupton, D. (1996) *The New Public Health: Health and Self in the Age of Risk*. London: Sage.

The VOICE Group (2010) 'Buying into motherhood? Problematic consumption and ambivalence in transitional phases'. *Consumption Markets & Culture*, 13: 373–397.

Wolf, J. (2011) *Is Breast Best? Taking on the Breastfeeding Experts and the New High Stakes of Motherhood*. New York and London: New York University Press.

Part 1

School and childcare settings

Chapter 2

Unsettling food encounters between families and early childhood educators

Deborah Albon

Introduction

Criticism of children's eating practices is commonplace in the UK and is enmeshed with ideas about foods considered to be 'proper' (or 'improper') as well as 'specific moralities about how family life should be' (Curtis et al., 2011: 65). This is a major theme circulating throughout this volume, which brings together papers offering a critical perspective on feeding children as a *social* practice rather than papers focused on children's nutritional intake. On entering school, family practices around food and eating become subject to the gaze of professionals, with school lunch boxes, for example, receiving particular attention in the literature in this respect (see e.g. Allison, 1991; Harman and Cappellini, 2015 and in this volume). Whilst the early childhood literature is replete with writing about 'good practice' in relation to food and eating (see e.g. Goldschmeid and Jackson, 1994; Manning-Morton and Thorp, 2003, as well as my own writing on the topic: Albon and Mukherji, 2008) I intend to use this paper to offer a detailed and more 'critical' examination of the gendered, classed and raced encounters which occur between families and early childhood educators in relation to food.

I suggest that a focus on 'early childhood' is of particular value at the current time because early childhood settings are often the first (regular) public space outside of the home that a young child encounters (Ben-Ari, 1997). Moreover, in public policy, nationally and internationally, early childhood settings are increasingly regarded as a panacea for an ever-widening assortment of social problems (Gulløv, 2012; see also Donovan et al., this volume). As Burman (1994: 172) has argued, early childhood settings/ schools have become 'the route to intervene in and reform family life' and governments' commitment to 'supporting' parents is 'driven by a particular moral agenda that seeks to regulate and control the behaviour of marginalized families' (Gillies, 2005: 71). One such area of regulation, I would argue, is families' food practices as there is an expectation that in early childhood young children will be inculcated into culturally inscribed 'rules' of what to eat and how to eat it (Ben-Ari, 1997).

In this chapter, I have chosen to present data relating to three areas which receive less attention in the literature on food practices in early childhood and/or school settings. First, I analyze the way that children's ability to 'eat nicely' in the early childhood setting they attend conjures particular perceptions of family life on the part of educators, which in turn serve to (further) marginalize some groups of families. Second, I present data related to children bringing in breakfast 'on the go' and constructions of the 'chaotic' family. And finally, I consider the 'fussy' mother/parent via a less usual instance of a mother who chose to bring in a hot meal from home each day. In drawing on data from two contrasting early childhood settings – a private day nursery and a nursery class attached to a primary school – I aim to show that the differing contexts of the settings impact markedly on the degree to which families are pathologized for their mealtime practices.

Before discussion of the methodology and data, I present an analysis of early childhood settings as 'civilizing' institutions including some brief historical context setting. 'Proper' mealtime practices will be shown to be a characteristic of the 'civilized' person and these are intertwined with middle class 'ideals' around the 'family meal' (Jackson, 2009), which are replicated in early childhood practice. I employ the term 'food event' throughout this paper as it is useful in including 'unstructured' times when food is eaten such as a snack on the move, which will be seen in discussion of eating breakfast 'on the go', as well as more 'structured' occasions such as mealtimes (Douglas and Nicod, 1974).

The early childhood context: institutions for 'civilizing' the body

Amongst a range of often competing, yet recurring, discourses of childhood: as a time of 'social investment', 'innocence' or 'vulnerability' to name but a few (Kirby and Woodhead, 2003), the idea that young children are 'uncivilized' or 'less civilized' than older (adult) human beings is pervasive (Shallwani, 2010; Albon and Hellman, 2018). It is generally parents who are charged with the job of 'civilizing' children (Elias, 1994; 1998), whose bodies are conceptualized variously, and often problematically, as 'unruly' and 'uncontrollable' (Grosz, 1994; Tobin, 1997) as well as 'malleable' and 'in need of discipline' (Leavitt and Power, 1997). But alongside parents, early childhood settings are similarly charged with supporting in this task in order to 'prepare' the child for school and for social life more generally. Early childhood educators are expected to work in 'partnership' with families, which in the English context is enshrined in statutory documentation such as the Early Years Foundation Stage (DfE, 2014). With 'partnership' in mind, Bach (2014) employs the term a 'concerted civilizing process' to denote the way that parents and educators are expected to work together in 'producing' the 'civilized' child (see also Truninger and Sousa, this volume).

The intervention of early childhood settings in family life has a long history. Gilliam and Gulløv (2014) argue that early childhood institutions developed in order to exercise control over the civilizing of the upcoming generation: in other words early childhood settings can be thought of as 'civilizing institutions.' According to their analysis, over time, children have come to be seen as requiring additional welfare provision outside the home alongside extended periods of economic dependency. To this end, children came to spend progressively more time outside the home in increasingly professionalized settings and in so doing they were subject to learning skills and behaviours deemed as 'civilized'. In terms of class relations, it was the upper classes who promoted the development of 'civilized' behaviour and 'civilized' communities in and outside early childhood settings with provision directed towards those of working-class backgrounds.

Early childhood settings are often the first, regular public space outside of the home that a young child encounters and can be viewed as interstitial in character in that they are charged with 'managing the movement of the child from the family into the "wider world"' (Ben-Ari, 1997: 96). In some settings, children receive breakfast, lunch and tea as well as snacks, 5 days a week for 50 weeks a year, and the 'early years' are seen as important in terms of nutrition but also in ensuring children inculcate 'good' eating habits which – it is suggested – will remain into adulthood (Children's Food Trust, 2012). Thus, 'food events' are of special import as they are an arena in which culturally inscribed 'rules' of behaviour – what to eat and how to eat it – are inculcated (Ben-Ari, 1997). Moreover, the cultivation of a particular set of cultural 'rules' pertaining to table manners (and display of them) can be viewed as emblematic of the 'civilized' person (Elias, 1994).

From its inception, the provision of meals for children in England was intertwined with instilling 'proper' modes of behaviour. A brief detour into the history of meals' provisioning for children in UK schools is perhaps productive at this point. Crowley and Cuff (1907), in the City of Bradford Education Committee Report on a Course of Meals given to Necessitous Children from April to July, 1907, reported on a feeding experiment carried out on about 40 children who were mostly from poor families. They noted the following:

> Every effort was made to make the meals, as far as possible, educational. There were tablecloths and flowers on the tables; monitresses, whose duty it was to lay the tables and to wait on the other children, were appointed … From almost the first there was very little to complain of in the general behaviours of the children, for children soon respond to orderly and decent surroundings. The table cloths, it is true were very dirty at the end of the week, but this was chiefly due to the dirty clothing of the children, and owing to the very inadequate provision at the school for the children to wash themselves, it was difficult to ensure that even their hands were clean.

Similarly, when children were not keen on the recipes (when much thought had been given to the menus), the report suggested:

> It is true that many of the meals suggested are not such as one is accustomed to find in the ordinary cottage home, and it might be objected that some of them involve too much thought and time to be used in the homes of the children. It would seem, however, that if such be the case, the fault lies with the upbringing of, and with the conditions under which many of the people live, rather than with the recipes.

In both instances working class families were seen as 'deficient' in terms of the cleanliness of the children and in the upbringing of their children. Moreover, children were viewed as responsive to the 'orderly and decent surroundings' of the table: the phrase infused with notions of class as well as notions of the school (and I would broaden this to include early childhood education and care) as a redemptive force (Penn, 2002; Osgood, 2012). What is clear, is that the public provision of meals was interwoven with class-based ideas of 'proper eating' and the (in)ability of working class families to feed their families 'properly'.

Even today, early childhood and school settings are expected to inculcate 'good' table manners alongside providing a meal. A recent OfSTED report EY288166 (one of many similar) states: 'They [the nursery children] sit well at the table and have excellent table manners, with older children reminding the younger ones about what is required.' Similarly, advertisements for school meals' supervisory assistants will ask for ability to assist in development of (or guidance on) table manners in job descriptions. Indeed, it is taken as 'given' that institutions such as nurseries and schools will inculcate 'good' table manners and social development more generally (Gilliam and Gulløv, 2014). In learning self-restraint and encouraging children to cooperate as a group (as together in close proximity), Gilliam and Gulløv (2014) view the EC setting – in an Eliasian sense – as an 'integration laboratory' (p. 15) in which children learn to develop behaviours towards others which are culturally 'acceptable' which they will carry forward into adulthood. As most children attend such institutions, they are subject to dominant notions of 'correct' behaviours and these come to be seen as 'ideal' conduct. According to Elias (1994), the child internalizes 'civilized' behaviours enabling him or her to integrate into the society within s/he resides.

Eating 'as a family' or, to employ the terminology often used in English early childhood settings: in small 'key groups' of children with an educator (Manning-Morton and Thorp, 2003), is often viewed as a prime means through which culturally accepted 'rules' of behaviour are expected to be modelled and replicated (see e.g. Children's Food Trust [2012] voluntary EY code of practice in *'Eat Better Start Better'*). As with ideas about the 'family meal', which is regarded as an important way in which families display or 'do' family (James and Curtis, 2010), English early childhood settings generally organize mealtime provisioning to resemble an idealized 'family style' mode of eating, embodied in the practice of sitting around a table in small groups, eating the same meal together. Yet evidence suggests that such mealtime practices were not universally adhered to historically in families, albeit that they have become symbolic of idealized family life (Murcott, 1997). And in recent times the 'family meal' may have been impacted by ever more complex work and social patterns (O'Connell and Brannen, 2016).

Early childhood educators are often advised that their provision mirror or extend that which is learnt or practised in the home. Goldschmeid and Jackson (1994: 181), for example, emphasize the need to provide 'as much consistency and continuity between the child's two worlds' (the home and the nursery). Yet I suspect it very unlikely that any setting would organize its mealtime provisioning in such a way that the children eat seated on the sofa in front of the television, albeit that for many families (and educators too) this may be their usual cultural practice. Moreover, for some, a dining table could be regarded as a luxury in terms of cost and in terms of the space it takes up in a family's home if space is at a premium. As James and Curtis (2011: 1178) assert, 'feeding one's family well is a visible and public sign of good parenting' and as 'civilizing institutions', arguably early childhood institutions act as bastions of 'proper', 'civilized' behaviour (Gilliam and Gulløv, 2014).

Methodology

The data I will be drawing on comes from an ethnographic study in which I spent 2 terms (one day a week) in four early childhood settings in turn across 3 local authorities in inner and outer London. In total the research involved more than 500 hours of fieldwork (2007–2010). For the purposes of this paper I am going to draw upon data from two of these settings as they offer a contrast in terms of the communities they serve and the educators who work there, the purpose and organisation of the settings and linked to this, the kinds of food provisioning on offer.

Setting One is a nursery class (39 children aged 3–4 years) attached to a state primary school on an estate comprising of social housing in West London. The school serves an ethnically diverse population, with many of the families being new to residing in the UK. In addition, the majority of families are in receipt of Income Support (welfare payment). Evidence from various documentation in the setting (e.g. school brochure) highlight how it is explicit in its mission to 'narrow the gap' and 'improve the life chances of children' who are deemed disadvantaged. Children in Setting One are provided with a fruit or vegetable snack mid-way in the session and can bring in a drink from home or pay for a milk (or have a free milk if in receipt of Income Support). The educators at the time of the study comprised of two middle class, White-British women, who are trained teachers, and one working class, Black-Caribbean woman, who is a nursery nurse/assistant (NVQ3) and unlike the other educators, lives on the estate.

Setting Two is a fee paying, private Montessori nursery (children from 6 months–5 years who may or may not attend each day), which is part of a small chain of three Montessori nurseries. It is situated in a church building in central London, on the cusp of two very distinct areas: economically and in terms of ethnic diversity. The majority of the educators come from the local working-class, British-Bangladeshi population and are either Montessori trained educators or have an NVQ2 or 3 qualification. The families are middle-class and primarily white-British/European. The nursery mostly serves working families in well-paid employment (e.g. journalists) and children are offered breakfast, dinner, tea and snacks in-between each day. A 'selling point' of the nursery is that it offers filtered water, organic food and has its own chef. The additional cost this incurs means the nursery is expensive compared to other private sector provision in the area. Unlike Setting One, this setting is open most of the year, only closing for major holidays.

The key aim of the study was to examine 'food events' in the context of the everyday 'life' of these settings, focusing on how 'rules' relating to food and food practices were constructed and maintained. Employing an ethnographic approach facilitated a detailed examination of the commonplace – here 'food events' – amongst the usual activity of the setting (Buchbinder et al., 2006). As is typical in ethnographic research (Hammersley and Atkinson, 2007), the study employed extensive reflective field-notes and semi-structured and less formal interviewing with educators and children. Although the children's families were not the prime focus of the study (unless they stayed for part or all of the nursery sessions/days) I observed many instances of interactions between educators and families, notably at the beginning and ends of sessions or days when children were dropped off or picked up from the nurseries, as well as noting many references to families in the interview data with educators.

For the purposes of this paper, I aim to highlight three themes which emerged from the data. In each case the emphasis is on how the home is made visible via food events. The first theme explores how family practices are 'writ large' on the bodies of young children as they display the degree to which they have learnt to 'eat nicely'. The second theme examines how children bringing in breakfast 'on the go' similarly serves as a lens through which educators make judgements about family life. The final theme examines data relating to a mother, who chose to bring in a hot meal from home and how this practice was perceived by educators. In each instance, I contrast the practice of the two early childhood settings.

The home made 'visible': children's ability to 'eat nicely'

In Setting One in particular, the ability of children to 'eat nicely' was viewed by educators as a lens through which to examine and comment upon family life. A typical example of this came during a snack time, which was a food event invariably held in the small kitchen space as opposed to the (larger) general nursery space. This was justified as being conducive to better hygiene as water was on hand to wipe children as needed, it was near to the bathroom, and because the space contained no soft furnishing or carpet that would be difficult to clean. The space was hugely at variance with the comfortable furnishing and plethora of equipment designed with young children in mind in the main area of the setting and seemed to represent a view of the child as 'uncivilized' (needing to be wiped, cleaned, contained, and controlled). Vera (a White, British, middle class educator) was describing why there had been a shift in the practice at snack times to having whole, unpeeled fruit on the table rather than segments or small pieces, which had been peeled/cut beforehand by the educators. When interviewed, she stated:

> Some children haven't learnt manners about food at home .... Now they see the whole fruit and it means snotty hands don't grab fruit and put it back on the plate – you know – when hands have gone in ... to be honest it puts you off eating the food yourself.

In her comment that some children 'haven't learnt manners' it was made explicit that these 'manners' should have been learnt in the home and replicated in the different context of the nursery classroom. And the expectation of 'manners' in instances such as this mirrors very directly the work of Elias (1994) as the ability to discipline the body and defer gratification for a while has come to be viewed in the English cultural context as 'good manners'. Moreover, the ability to maintain bodily separateness has also come to be regarded as a vital characteristic of the 'civilized' person.

In this setting, ideas about 'good manners' often permeated discussion about children and families and children's 'performances' at the table served to make the home visible to educators. In the following interaction, the children had some salad vegetables to eat which had been grown in the school garden.

> Duane (a Black, working class boy aged 3 years) picks up salad with his fingers. Mary (a White, middle class educator) admonishes him, saying publicly and 'jokingly': 'were you born in a barn Duane? Use your knife and fork.'

The colloquial reference to being 'born in a barn', although said in a 'jocular' fashion, served to pathologize Duane and his family yet this same educator confided examples of practice in the dining hall when the children moved through to the reception class where she had stepped in to challenge practice she'd observed. In one notable example, Mary asserted:

> One of the Dinner Ladies said to one of the Asian children 'don't they teach you to eat properly at home' when the child was using her cup of water to wash her fingers – she had been picking up her food with her fingers – I had to have a word with her to tell her that's what *they* do.

Perhaps Mary was keen that I should see her in a positive light in sharing this story, but her phrase: 'what *they* do' (the italics mirroring her emphasis of this word) positioned Asian families as Other to the White, middle class majority of staff (not families) in the school. Moreover, it assumed food-related cultural practices as homogenous to Asian families as a whole.

In setting two I observed no such admonishing of parents for their children's supposed 'lack' of table manners, despite the fact that the children were more 'on show' in this regard than in setting one as the children ate breakfast, lunch and tea in the setting with snacks in-between. A number of possible explanations can be offered here: The children in this setting were spread across the 6 month–5 years age-range and there was, understandably, less expectation that the very youngest babies/children in this age-range would have learnt such behaviours and be able to reproduce them. Furthermore, the families in this setting were White and middle class, unlike the educators and this coupled with the dynamic of working in a for-profit nursery, which had a focus on supporting working families, impacted on the relationships between families and educators (see also Osgood, 2005; 2012). The raison d'etre of the setting was not to 'compensate' for a supposed 'lack' in the children's home lives, which has a long history in public sector nursery provision (Whitbread, 1972): indeed I never once heard families criticized for their food practices – a point I develop in more detail later. I did, however, see similar expectations and modelling by educators in both settings around 'civilized' mealtime behaviour in their interactions with children at the table. The key difference was that in Setting Two, the 'uncivilized' table manners of the children, such as grabbing food from a plate before having it offered or smearing food onto their bodies, was solely put down to their younger age and not related to the social class of their families.

A further point of interest here is that the central assumption that circulates throughout this theme is that children passively reproduce particular practices from the home in the school or nursery setting (Grieshaber, 2004), rather than (perhaps) behaving differently in the different social context or indeed shifting their behaviour as a result of interactions with the peer group (Albon and Hellman, 2018). I saw many examples of children (in the 2–5 years age range) engaged in activity such as surreptitiously smearing soft foods such as banana onto their tummies, or waiting until an educator's back was turned and showing each other the masticated food within their mouths. The hiding of such practices suggests that these children were well aware that these behaviours were outside normative ideas of 'civilized' behaviour, but nonetheless delighted in behaving otherwise. On other occasions I observed examples of children reinforcing the rules such as 'ratting' on those whose behaviour was 'outside' the norms of the setting. Thus, it is simplistic to imagine children passively reproduce the food practices of their home in the school context (or indeed vice versa) and indicates that peer relations play an important part in food events in early childhood settings (Albon and Hellman, 2018).

The home made 'visible': bringing breakfast in from home

My focus now shifts to a food-related activity which receives little attention in the literature: instances when children bring in breakfast from home, perhaps eating it as they arrive in the setting. This was a practice I observed in both settings, and, I will argue, was illustrative of the way class relations played out in each context.

On most of the days when I was present in Setting One, one or more children (of the 39 on roll) would arrive in the process of eating. Generally, these children were bundled by educators into the kitchen area, which was separated off from the main nursery classroom, but was a visible space via a stable-door. Sometimes, this separating off of the children was accompanied by exaggerated sighs of disapproval or comments, which on the surface were directed at children such as 'you haven't finished your breakfast *before* nursery AGAIN' (Charmagne, Black working class educator, setting one). But these comments/sighs/ separations from the main room were directed as much towards the parent(s) as the child albeit that the educator's exaggerated tone of voice 'signalled' that they were talking to the child. The 'message' to parents and their children seemed to state firmly that the main 'business' of the nursery was not to ensure the children were fed but to educate the children. And the separation from the main room acted as a geographical reminder – if one was needed – that bringing in breakfast from home was a practice that was Other to that expected from families using the nursery.

It is worth commenting that Charmagne was a Black, working class lone parent with children who attended the school where she worked. She lived locally on the estate and often tried to distance herself from working class families deemed 'chaotic' by the educator team. The work of Osgood (2012) is useful here in highlighting how some working class women who become early childhood educators attempt to construct a professional identity for themselves which is distinct – even superior – to that of their working class counterparts and this seemed evident in my discussions with Charmagne, who would often juxtapose her own 'better' food practices compared to those of some of the families she worked with.

The exasperation each of the educators felt about children arriving with breakfast part-eaten is also exemplified in the following interview extract when Kelly (a White, middle class educator in Setting One) noted:

> I'll tell you what I find really hard here – when you see some of the children coming into nursery, clutching what they've had for breakfast and it's something that is totally inappropriate, like a muffin, or a cupcake, or a bag of crisps, or half a waffle. I don't think I've ever seen anyone come in with anything that is even remotely appropriate to have for breakfast. It just smacks of being disorganised.

On the one hand, Kelly seems to profess that there is universal agreement about the food stuffs deemed 'appropriate' for breakfast time. She also uses the phrase 'it just smacks of being disorganised' to describe the way some children had not eaten or finished eating their breakfast at home. Curtis et al. (2011) argue there is a great deal of moralizing around particular foods and food practices and how these 'fit' with notions of 'proper' family life and a 'proper' family practice would be to ensure meals are finished at home prior to coming to nursery/school. Yet many of these families had to get a number of children ready for nursery/school, including being fed, in a context where lateness was frowned and subject to external scrutiny. The national regulatory body: OfSTED, for example, reports on a wide range of activity in schools including attendance and punctuality.

Families in Setting One did not verbally challenge the admonishments of the educators as far as I observed. Some seemed to directly ignore the criticism, allowing it to 'wash over' them seemingly unregistered and other parents adopted a strategy, deliberate or unintentional, of pre-empting potential reprimand through a great deal of apologising, perhaps over and above the 'crime' of bringing in breakfast. I saw repeated examples of bringing in breakfast 'on the go' from some families so the chastisements they endured did not seem to change their behaviour.

Children were seen to arrive in the midst of eating breakfast in Setting Two too, even though families could choose (but pay extra) to have breakfast provided by the nursery. However, these children (and by association their families) were not separated off from the group. In part this was geographical as the rooms were very small and had no additional, visible space such as a kitchen attached to them: the kitchen was an entirely separate space serving the entire nursery via individual trolleys per room. Children eating on arrival were asked to sit somewhere alongside the group to finish their breakfast and the educators went out of their way to help the parents settle their child swiftly enabling them to go to work, saying e.g. 'don't worry I will make sure he finishes his toast', helping take off coats etc ... to aid parents. Most parents seemed to be in a rush in this setting, often citing deadlines for their journalistic copy or important meetings as explanation for their 'disorganisation'. Nadiya (a British-Bangladeshi, working class educator in Setting Two) stated:

> It can be difficult for them (i.e. parents organising breakfast for their children). They have really good jobs – some are journalists – and they work long hours.

In these two examples, 'chaos' was differently constructed according to the social class and perceived work patterns of the families. As Gillies (2005: 85) has argued '"Good" parents are constructed as resourceful, agentic and ethically responsible, able to recognize or learn what is best for their children and tailor their behaviour accordingly'. The middle class, White parents in Setting Two were able to employ 'throw-away' references to their professional roles as a resource through which to position their 'disorganisation' and need of help. And in so doing they were able to 'trump' the professionalism of the working class, Bangladeshi/British early childhood educators who unfailingly (in my fieldwork) deferred to them and supported them. Unlike the families in Setting One, these families were not constructed as needing 'educating' in relation to food practices, which seemed to have its basis in their (middle) social class and because they were mostly working in well-paid, well-regarded professions. However, the picture is more complex as I would argue that differentials between the two settings is interwoven with the type of provision the children attend– a point I take up in more detail in the final discussion.

The home made 'visible': bringing hot food in from home at lunchtime

It was rare in both settings for children to bring in a main meal from home. Some children in Setting One did bring in a packed lunch once reaching the reception class where they ate alongside older children on long benches in a large dining hall. On many occasions I heard educators talk about the 'quality' of food in children's lunchboxes in terms of hygiene and the nutritional content of the food, but here I wish to focus on a less usual exemplar: a mother who brought in a hot meal from home every lunchtime. My fieldnotes state:

> Ashu has just entered the reception class from the nursery and his mother comes in each day with a hot meal at lunch-time. So he does not have a cold packed lunch nor does he have the school dinner. This causes much consternation amongst the staff.

Children who bought in a cold packed lunch put their lunchbox into a shared storage box in their classroom at the beginning of the day, which was wheeled round to the dining hall at lunchtime. This fitted in with the institutional organisation of the school unlike bringing in a hot meal from home. Ashu's mother came in every day, just before lunchtime, and handed over a hot meal of freshly prepared chapati, dhal, and vegetables to the school reception desk staff. Clearly a lot of effort had gone into preparing this and a fresh linen napkin was always included with the meal.

Jo (White, middle class educator) in Setting One argued:

> She cannot expect us to let her do this forever. She's way too fussy and this is why Ashu is the way he is.

Further context setting sheds more light on this data as Ashu had recently moved to the reception class of the school from the nursery and each morning was generally regarded by the educators as reluctant to leave his mother, crying for long periods when she left. The comment from Jo that 'this is why [he] is the way he is' links to Ashu's behaviour beyond mealtimes, which was regarded as problematic: a child unable to separate from his mother 'successfully'.

Cairns et al., in this volume, discuss how mothers' feeding practices are stigmatized if at the extremes of 'bad mom' and 'obsessed mom' and this is mirrored in this research. Unlike the 'chaotic' families in the breakfast exemplars in the previous section, in the extract above we see a quite different but nonetheless 'problematic' view of the home/mothering – the 'overly protective' or 'fussy' mother. Yet the preparation and presentation of the food and the accompanying linen napkin seemed the very embodiment of 'civility'. This was a school where predominantly the staff were white and British and this was a mother who was born in South India, and although not stated explicitly, the educators seemed to equate her 'fussiness' with her ethnic background. To expand, this mother's parenting was constructed as 'unhelpful' in supporting her child to become 'independent', which is a dominant discourse in Western culture (Shallwani, 2010) – particularly on entry to school. By way of contrast, the pleasure to be derived from lovingly preparing food for one's own child and the inter-dependence this engenders (see Siraj-Blatchford and Clarke, 2000) was frowned upon.

Ashu was regarded as having his mother 'wrapped round his little finger' (Mary, Setting One) and his mother was viewed as being very submissive to his and her family's demands. An alternative explanation, I suggest, is that this mother strongly challenged the food practices of this school in insisting that Ashu had a hot meal prepared by her. She never apologized for bringing in the hot food as far as I could ascertain and for the duration that I was in the setting (two terms) continued to do this. A major concern expressed by educators was that it would result in a 'slippery slope' of others following this practice, but this did not materialize during my time of fieldwork.

In Setting Two, I saw no instances of families bringing in a hot meal from home but I did observe instances of 'tasting evenings' which were occasions when parents could come to discuss menus, try new recipes, and ask questions of the owner and chef as to the food provisioning or raise issues such as food intolerances and allergies. The provision of locally sourced food as well as organic produce were a passion of the owner and were a distinct marketing ploy used to 'sell' the setting to middle class families. The middle class parents who attended such sessions were not considered 'fussy', unlike the mother in Setting One above, but were seen as exercising their right to demand a particular service. Their desires for particular foods were generally listened to and acted upon, but the mismatch between the practice of the setting and the educators' experience away from the setting was palpable, with Shaheen (a British, Bangladeshi educator) telling me in hushed tones in the staff room one day: 'we don't feed *our* children this food [talking about the educators' own children and not those of the families she worked with] but these families *expect* it and you've got to be very, very careful.' In part, I think she was fearful of criticising families who were significant in her retaining employment; although she was not paid much more than the minimum wage (unlike the parents' employment), hers was the prime wage for her family.

Discussion

The data suggest divergence between the two settings in terms of gendered, classed and raced food encounters between early childhood educators and families. But this begs the question: why? I now wish to tease out some possible explanations.

First, all families who used Setting Two were White British or European/ middle-class and those who worked were in well-paid employment. The differential in the families' homes in comparison to the educators was stark as the families tended to live in large houses or apartments converted from old warehouses along the Thames, which are incredibly expensive and out of reach for an early childhood workforce receiving the minimum wage for caring for their children. Most of the educators lived in social housing. Indeed on one occasion I observed a father showing one of the educators the specification of a Thames-side flat he was about to view and noted a price-tag of over £2,000,000. Although this was a gesture of 'familiarity' towards his child's caregiver in the nursery it felt an uncomfortable encounter as the educator would never be able to afford such a home. Differentials in the class background, ethnicity and wealth of the educators seemed to result in deference towards parents akin to servitude that was not seen in Setting One where two of the three educators (and the lead educators in the setting) were White, British and middle class unlike the majority of families (see Osgood, 2012; Vincent and Ball, 2006). Harman and Cappellini's work, in this volume, similarly highlights the intersection of ethnicity, gender and social class in relation to families' foodwork – with a focus on lunchboxes – arguing that lunchboxes are replete with cultural complexity and are subject to scrutiny by settings.

Second, the type of early childhood provision is of significance. Setting One is a free service (a nursery class attached to a school) in the public sector on an estate comprising social housing, whereas Setting Two is a private sector nursery, serving an affluent population. The *raison d'etre* of each provision is very different and there has long been a view of public nursery education's 'redemptive' role in compensating for supposed deficiencies in the home by replicating middle class child-rearing practices (James, 2012). By way of contrast, the private sector nursery in the study is very expensive and as such, is in an explicitly financial relationship with families which can perhaps be best summed up as 'the customer is always right'. Thus, the *raison d'etre* of a given setting or set of provisions is entwined with the goals of its feeding programmes: an issue which is picked up later by Donovan et al., in this volume.

Finally, the settings also differed in the kind of provision on offer, highlighting long-held divisions between care and education in early childhood provision (James, 2012). Being part of a school meant that Setting One had an explicitly 'educational' agenda, whereas Setting Two clearly offered a combination of care and education, not least evidenced in the number of 'food events' the children participated in during the day and the hours of availability (with few closure days) of the setting. Linked to this, the professional background of the educators differed markedly too, as in Setting One, two of the educators had been trained as teachers and one as a nursery nurse/assistant, whereas no educator held a teaching certificate beyond a Montessori Diploma in Setting Two. These variations in professional background may also offer insight into the contrast between the two settings, for example some teacher-trained educators may not view the 'purpose' of their role as supporting families and ensuring children are well-fed.

Conclusion

The evidence from this study is that food events constitute occasions when the home/family life is made 'visible' to early childhood educators. The data show that issues of class, ethnicity and gender permeate encounters in early childhood settings, not least in relation to what constitutes 'proper' family practices in relation to food. Although sometimes considered to be 'civilizing institutions' (Gilliam and Gulløv, 2014), young children and their families display a range of strategies to resist and subvert what might be regarded as the '*over* civilizing' (Leavitt and Power, 1997) practices of the early childhood setting they attended. Indeed attempts at moderating the food practices of parents in Setting One were largely ignored and unthinkable in Setting

Two. The construction of the young child as 'malleable' perhaps encourages a shared belief in the young child's body as more 'receptive' than adults to the 'civilizing processes' employed in and around food events. This is an area worthy of greater interrogation but beyond the purview of this present paper.

Here, I sought to highlight a complex interplay of factors which infuse food encounters between early childhood educators and families such as social class, race, gender and employment type. For profit, private early childhood settings have a very different relationship with families than that of the public sector, with primarily working class women providing care for middle class women – an inverse of middle class women providing education for working class families, as in many school settings (Osgood, 2005; 2012). Rather than having a 'redemptive' or 'compensatory' view of their role, such settings are embedded in a context where market relations dominate. The data presented here represents two 'extremes', with *neither* context making for 'comfortable' food encounters between educators and families. The picture which emerges is one which unsettles the notion of 'partnership' between early childhood settings and families and it is precisely for this reason that I would argue further examination of 'food events' is needed as it can offer a valuable lens through which to consider encounters between early childhood educators and families more broadly.

References

Albon, D. and Hellman, A. (2018). 'Of Routine Consideration: "Civilising" Children's Bodies via Food Events in Swedish and English Early Childhood Settings'. *Ethnography and Education*, published online 10. 1. 18, DOI: 10.1080/17457823. 2017.1422985. 1–16.

Albon, D. and Mukherji, P. (2008). *Food and Health in Early Childhood*, London: Sage.

Allison, A. (1991) 'Japanese Mothers and Obentos: The Lunch-box as Ideological State Apparatus', *Anthropological Quarterly*, 64(4): 195–208.

Bach, D. (2014). 'Parenting Among Wealthy Danish families: A Concerted Civilising Process', *Ethnography and Education*, 9(2): 224–237.

Ben-Ari, E. (1997). *Body Projects in Japanese Childcare: Culture, Organization and Emotions in a Preschool*, Richmond: Curzon Press.

Buchbinder, M., Longhofer, J., Barrett, T., Lawson, P. and Floersch, J. (2006). 'Ethnographic Approaches to Child Care Research', *Journal of Early Childhood Research*, 4(1): 45–63.

Burman, E. (1994). *Deconstructing Developmental Psychology*, London: Routledge.

Children's Food Trust (2012). *Eat Better Start Better*, Sheffield: Children's Food Trust, www.childrensfoodtrust.org.uk (accessed 12. 10. 16).

Crowley, R.H. (Medical Superintendent) in conjunction with Cuff, M.E. (Superintendent of Domestic Subjects) (1907). City of Bradford Education Committee Report on a Course of Meals given to Necessitous Children from April to July, 1907. From National Archives online.

Curtis, P., James, A. and Ellis, K. (2011). 'Children's Snacking, Children's Food: Food Moralities and Family Life', in S. Punch, I. McIntosh, R. Edmond (Eds) *Children's Food Practices in Families and Institutions*, Abingdon: Routledge. (pp. 65–76).

Department for Education (2014). *Statutory Framework for The Early Years Foundation Stage*, Nottingham: DfE.

Douglas, M. and Nicod, M. (1974). 'Taking the Biscuit: The Structure of British Meals', *New Society*, 30(637): 744–747.

Elias, N. (1994). *The Civilizing Process*, Oxford: Blackwell.

Elias, N. (1998). 'The Civilizing of Parents', in J. Gouldsblom and S. Mennell (Eds) *The Norbert Elias Reader*, Oxford: Blackwell. (pp. 189–211).

Gilliam, L. and Gulløv, E. (2014). 'Making Children "Social": Civilizing Institutions in the Danish Welfare State', *Human Figurations*, 3(1): 1–20. http://hdl.handle.net/2027/spo.11217607.0003.103 (accessed 20. 10. 16).

Gillies, V. (2005). 'Meeting Parents' Needs? Discourses of "Support" and "Inclusion" in Family Policy', *Critical Social Policy*, 25(1): 70–90.

Goldschmeid, E. and Jackson, S. (1994). *People Under Three: Young Children in Day care*, London: Routledge.

Grieshaber, S. (2004). *Rethinking Parent and Child Conflict*. London: Routledge/Falmer.

Grosz, E. (1994). *Volatile Bodies: Toward a Corporeal Feminism*. Bloomington: Indiana University Press.

Gulløv, E. (2012). 'Kindergartens in Denmark: Reflections on Continuity and Change', in A.T Kjørholt and J. Qvortrup (Eds) *The Modern Child and the Flexible Labour Market. Studies in Childhood and Youth*. London:Palgrave Macmillan. (pp. 90–107).

Hammersley, M. and Atkinson, P. (2007). *Ethnography: Principles in Practice* (3rd ed), Abingdon: Routledge.

Harman, V. and Cappellini, B. (2015). 'Mothers on Display: Lunchboxes, Social Class and Moral Accountability', *Sociology*, 49(4): 764–781.

Jackson, P. (2009). 'Introduction: Food a Lens on Family Life', in P. Jackson (Ed.) *Changing Families, Changing Food*. London: Palgrave Macmillan. (pp. 1–16).

James, A. (2012). 'Child-Centredness and the "Child": The Cultural Politics of Nursery Schooling in England', in A.T. Kjorholt and J. Quortrup (Eds), *The Modern Child and the Flexible Labour Market*. London: Palgrave Macmillan. (pp 111–127).

James, A. and Curtis, P. (2010) 'Family Displays and Personal Lives', *Sociology*, 44(6): 1163–1180.

Kirby, P. and Woodhead, M. (2003). 'Children's Participation in Society', in H. Montgomery, R. Burr, and M. Woodhead (Eds) *Changing Childhoods: Local and Global*, Milton Keynes: OUP. (pp. 233–284).

Leavitt, R. and Power, M.B. (1997). 'Civilizing Bodies: Children in Day Care', in J. Tobin (Ed.), *Making a Place for Pleasure in Early Childhood Education*, New Haven and London: Yale University Press. (pp. 39–75).

Manning-Morton, J. and Thorp, M. (2003). *Key Times for Play*, Maidenhead: OUP.

Murcott, A. (1997). 'Family Meals – A Thing of the Past?' in P. Caplan (Ed.) *Food, Identity and Health*, London: Routledge. (pp. 32–49).

O'Connell, R. and Brannen, J. (2016). *Food, Families and Work*, London: Bloomsbury.

Osgood, J. (2005). 'Who cares? The Classed Nature of Childcare', *Gender and Education*, 17(3): 289–303.

Osgood, J. (2012). *Narratives from the Nursery: Negotiating Professional Identities in Early Childhood*, London: Routledge.

Penn, H. (2002). 'The World Bank's View of Early Childhood', *Childhood*, 9(1): 118–132.
Shallwani, S. (2010). 'Racism and Imperialism in Child Development Discourse: Deconstructing 'Developmentally Appropriate Practice', in G.S. Cannella, L. Diaz Soto (Eds) *Childhoods: A Handbook*, New York: Peter Lang. (pp. 231–244).
Siraj-Blatchford, I. and Clarke, P. (2000). *Supporting Identity, Diversity and Language in the Early Years*, Buckingham: OUP.
Tobin, J. (1997). 'Introduction: The Missing Discourse of Pleasure and Desire', in J. Tobin (Ed.), *Making a Place for Pleasure in Early Childhood Education*. New Haven: Yale University Press. (pp. 1–37).
Vincent, C. and Ball, S.J. (2006). *Childcare, Choice and Class Practices*, London: Taylor and Francis.
Whitbread, N. (1972). *The Evolution of the Nursery-Infant School*, London: Routledge and Kegan Paul.

Chapter 3

Intersectionality and migrant parents' perspectives on preparing lunchboxes for their children

Vicki Harman and Benedetta Cappellini

Introduction

Food work operates within a wider context including demographic, cultural, social and technological factors. As part of this, migration and mobilities have influenced people's practices and the context in which they make food-related decisions. Vertovec (2007) employs the term 'super-diversity' to refer to the level and complexity of contemporary diversity in Britain and argues that this is particularly visible in London. When seeking to understand the experiences of migrants a range of factors need to be taken into account, including country of origin, migration channel, language and area of residence. In 2001, the then Foreign Secretary in Britain, Robin Cook declared that 'Chicken tikka masala is now a true British national dish, not only because it is the most popular, but because it is a perfect illustration of the way Britain absorbs and adapts external influences' (*The Guardian*, 19.04.01). Hybridity visible within food practices can be positively regarded as emblematic of multiculturalism in action or it can be regarded with suspicion, linking to fears of loss of cultural traditions and concerns about authenticity (Pitcher, 2014).

Focusing on parents' perspectives, this chapter explores lunchboxes as a site of everyday care for children. Lunchboxes are significant because they are communicative: as domestic food going outside of the home they convey not only love and care for children but also aspects of the family's ethnic identity and social position. This chapter asks: How far can intersectionality be a useful term when examining parents' perspectives on preparing lunchboxes for their children? How salient are migration and ethnicity within migrant parents' narratives of preparing lunchboxes for their children? Are other identities such as social class and gender equally or more visible in their narratives?

Intersectionality has been a key term put forward by feminist scholars in order to promote an understanding of the inter-related nature of structures of oppression. Kimberlé Crenshaw introduced the concept of intersectionality in 1989 when discussing black women's experiences with regard to employment (for more background and debate see Yuval-Davis, 2006). Black feminist scholars including bell hooks (1981) have highlighted how sexism intersects with racial stereotyping to doubly disadvantage black women. Scholars have built on this understanding through empirical research that highlights how social positions can confer both advantages and disadvantages. For example, Fathi (2017) examines the narratives of middle-class Iranian female doctors in the UK. By examining areas of belonging and areas where these women feel they do not belong, Fathi (2017) provides an understanding of how social class, ethnicity, migration and gender intersect.

In this chapter we understand ethnicity as referring to cultural markers of difference based on notions of nation, belonging, shared history and heritage (Garner, 2010). Connections between consumer behaviour, ethnicity and identity and belonging have been identified as important within academic scholarship (Venkatesh, 1995; Pitcher, 2014). Consumption can be an important vehicle through which ethnicity and status are expressed both in public and private, and a vehicle through which hybrid identities can be formed (Sekhon, 2007). Empirical studies concerning ethnicity and parenting have shown how families seek to pass cultural and religious practices down to the next generation, who may be living in a different environment to where parents were brought up as children (Barn, Ladino and Rogers, 2006; Becher, 2008; Hodges and Wiggins, 2013). Personal stories and current practices can therefore be intertwined with families' migrations and food histories, and both change and continuity in practices can be identified (see for example Alibhai-Brown, 2009; Cappellini and Yen, 2016). Yet food is also political and parents might be criticised for sticking too closely to traditional food patterns (see Albon, this volume). At the same time food cultures can become commodified, with the three S's of Samosas, Saris and Steel bands being emblematic of a stereotypical view of multiculturalism (Pitcher, 2014). The problem with this is that it seems to fix cultural practices in time and treat them as though they are somehow essential in their association with their participants. This does not adequately recognise how food practices might change as a result of acculturation, and the availability of different food types. For example, consumer research on immigrant mothers reveals how they negotiate their integration to their new cultural context via 'cultural swapping' (Oswald, 1999). Indeed, they display different identities depending on the situation, showing a greater integration to the 'host' culture in public contexts, while maintaining their 'home' culture in private contexts (Cappellini and Yen, 2016). In reserving food from their 'home country' for domestic consumption settings, while consuming 'mainstream' food in public contexts, these women show how food swapping practices are at play in their everyday lives. Able to accommodate the diet of their families depending on the situations, they show how food is central for maintaining their belonging to various cultures. Such practices intersect with social class (Skeggs, 2004) whereby middle- and upper- class individuals possess increased economic, cultural and social capitals enabling them to engage in these practices. As previous studies have shown, mothers often consider 'feeding the family' a duty central to their identity as a 'good' mother (DeVault, 1991). Described as a restless work in which love, fatigue, joy and anxieties collide, feeding the family is often seen as a way of teaching children about health, self-discipline, cosmopolitanism and 'good' taste. In contrast, for working class mothers, food work appears to be less about perpetuating privileges and more a matter of getting people fed and allowing children to make autonomous choices about their food (Wills et al., 2011).

Food work can also be communicative within the household as well as outside. For example, Chowbey's (2017) study of South Asian women in Britain, India and Pakistan found that women sometimes tried to negotiate more powerful positions within the household through food. Food practices, such as aligning one's diet with that of certain family members or refusing to cook or eat certain types of food favoured by others, could be a way of communicating conflict as well as love (Chowbey, 2017).

Lunchboxes and parenting: an overview of the literature

Critical studies looking at children's lunchboxes show how food in packed lunches 'is balanced, culturally rather than nutritionally' (Metcalfe et al., 2008: 405). Highlighting how the 'right' way of balancing food often reflects wider social and structural norms and conventions of other meals, studies show how the notion of 'good' food is culturally influenced. Social class is indeed a key element in influencing such a notion, as demonstrated by Donner (2006). Her study illustrates how middle-class Bengali women use discourses of hygiene and practicality surrounding the process of making a lunchbox in order to display social class outside home. Institutions such as schools can, through their promotion of 'good' food, support national discourses about belonging and earned/ active citizenship. For example, Karrebæk's (2012) study of lunchboxes in Denmark, demonstrates how school regulations sanctioning some foods while encouraging the consumption of others, is a way of disregarding the culinary cultures of ethnic minorities and re-establishing Danish cultural dominance. Insisting on the desirability of eating Danish bread – justified mainly in nutritional terms – school regulations reinforce the ideals of the superiority of the dominant culinary culture and provide an apparently 'neutral' justification for marginalising ethnic minorities. Similarly, Allison's (1991) paper based on her own experience of being an American mother making obento boxes for her child in Japan, shows how local school regulations promote specific ideals of meals, family life and motherhood. Indeed, 'good' mothering was judged as such if women conform to wider culinary conventions of aesthetically appealing and nutritious bento boxes. Deviating from such conventions was seen by the school as a sign of being a mother in need of attention and guidance of how to mother 'appropriately'.

Studies looking at the UK context have illustrated how media and politicised initiatives around healthy eating in schools (Hollows and Jones, 2010), and the organisation of time and space of lunch breaks (Daniel and Gustafsson, 2010; Metcalfe et al., 2008) can be viewed as tools of disciplining children and mothers (Pike, 2008). These studies show how school regulations around 'healthy eating' tend to promote a white and middle-class way of mothering and to stigmatise working-class mothers deviating from the dominant middle-class narratives of feeding children (Pike and Leahy, 2012). Relatedly, Vincent et al., (2012) discuss the strategies used by Black middle-class parents in England in relation to schools. One parent interviewed for their study described significant pressure to get the lunchbox 'right' in the context of the promotion of healthy eating at the current time. She was able to mobilise several capitals to meet this symbolically important task (Vincent et al., 2012). This was echoed in our own work, in which we highlighted how middle-class mothers are more confident in navigating school regulations and thus displaying good mothering outside the home. Working-class mothers tended to be less orchestrated in their public display of mothering and therefore may be more likely to come into conflict with school regulations (Cappellini, Harman and Parsons, 2018).

In our previous works (Harman and Cappellini, 2015; Harman and Cappellini, 2017), we have also highlighted how the lunchbox is embedded in gendered notions of 'good' and 'intensive' mothering. Preparing the perfect lunchbox is a never fully achieved task, as mothers feel that they need to constantly 'learn' and experiment with the new food items available on the market. Also, mothers often feel that they are the only ones in the family able to mediate between the market's offers, children's tastes and changing desires and school regulations (Harman and Cappellini, 2017). Such a mediation is a complex work of providing food considered nutritious and enjoyable for the children, also following the school's regulations of what constitutes a 'good' lunch. Indeed, providing leisure through food is a common practice amongst some participants who engage in elaborated preparation to entertain children and facilitate their eating (Harman and Cappellini, 2014). Others hide certain items (e.g. chocolate sweets) banned from the school, using them as 'treats' and rewards to their children. Respecting school regulations and pleasing children are not the only aims guiding women in their mundane task of preparing lunchboxes. Displaying good mothering to the self, to other family members and to other mothers is indeed a driving aim, informing the planning of lunchboxes (Harman and Cappellini, 2015). We seek to extend this understanding from the literature here by considering how lunchboxes might also reveal messages about parents' and children's ethnic identity as well as other social identities.

Research Methods

This study focuses on the narratives of parents who had migrated to England from other countries. They were drawn from a wider study of thirty one participants (thirty mothers and one father) interviewed between January 2013 and July 2014 plus three focus groups (nineteen participants in total) from the same group of parents. All participants lived in the South East of England, in London and Surrey.

Research participants were recruited via a letter sent out by schools to all parents with children aged 9–11 at their school. Parents with children aged between nine and eleven years old were targeted since children at this stage have well established food preferences and can negotiate their choices with adults (Roberts and Pettigrew, 2013).

Participants were interviewed twice. The first interview provided an introduction to each family, how food was organised within the household, responsibility for meals and shopping including preparing lunchboxes, how the lunchbox content was decided, and guidance given from the school and other sources. Parents were then asked to take photographs of lunchboxes prepared during one week. In the second interview, which took place after we received the photographs, parents were asked to reflect on their photographs and to discuss these with the interviewer. Ethnicity and migration were not areas of explicit focus within the interview guide, but rather emerged naturally from the conversation between interviewer and participant, as well as in the analysis.

The focus groups enabled participants to discuss lunchboxes in a group setting, facilitating the interactions between mothers with different experiences, ideas and understandings. Here, parents were shown photographs of lunchboxes and a recent news article as a stimulus for discussion. A thematic data analysis began after the first interview and was ongoing. For the purposes of this chapter, we focus on the interview narratives of three migrant parents, analysing how social identities can be read as being reflected in the lunchboxes they prepare.

Jasmeen's chapatis

Jasmeen is originally from India and lives in London with her 9 year old daughter and her husband. They live in a council flat located in a relatively wealthy urban area. Jasmeen's husband is a freelance chef and works long hours, while she works part time in a local supermarket. She considers the duty of 'taking care' of her family to belong to herself. Such a duty is mainly framed as a matter of providing 'good food' for her family, a practice that occupies the majority of Jasmeen's free time.

For Jasmeen, good food is defined as Indian food. Jasmeen explained that the type of food she prepares for her daughter is an important link to her cultural heritage as the food she prepares represents 'our typical lunchbox in India'. In her interview Jasmeen explained that she gets up at around 5am each morning to begin cooking (a process which takes 45 minutes to 1 hour). She described this as: 'Rush hour that time, busy time, morning'. But the mental preparation and aspects of the cooking have already begun the night before. She explained:

> Suppose I want to make spinach paratha. So first in the night time the previous day I'm making spinach curry, dough and everything I'm making ready, and morning I'm making the spinach paratha. The next day I'm thinking, 'Okay, I will give leftover curry with chapati.' So morning I'm making fresh chapati, and curry is left over from previous day.

When the cooking has been completed, she, her husband and her daughter generally eat this food for breakfast and following this she packs the rest for her daughter to eat at lunchtime. Sometimes, her daughter or husband will have cereal instead for breakfast. Jasmeen's consumption practices and the domestic work she puts into food preparation provide an important link to her country of origin which she is passing down to her daughter. She explained that:

> In my childhood, we used to eat chapati and one curry in India. Curry or dry curry, our typical lunchbox in India. In India people are eating like that. So I'm giving food on that basis, but making something more innovative or different things. [...] You know you have dosa in India, yellow mashed potato curry. That's the mashed potato curry but I add green peas, spinach and bread and I made like a cutlet.

Such 'innovations' are directed towards her daughter's taste preferences. In terms of the feelings associated with preparing lunchboxes, Jasmeen said that she does not always enjoy it: 'sometimes it's boring continuous cooking. That is life.' Furthermore she says that sometimes she feels angry because she comes home from work, tired, and has to go straight to the kitchen. However, she said 'as a mother, that is my job, she [her daughter] should be healthy because my mum gave me healthy food, that's why. You know green leaf vegetables.' As well as seeing this as mothers' work, Jasmeen also expressed pride in the knowledge that her daughter enjoyed the food that she had prepared more than the food provided by the school. According to this narrative, Jasmeen puts aside her own feelings to put her daughter's needs and interests first. Although she doesn't always enjoy all aspects of the labour, she is carried forward by the knowledge that her work is valued by her daughter and by herself. In addition to lunchboxes, Jasmeen talked about cooking food for school events which was served by her daughter to other children and their parents:

> Yesterday I made bhel in the school, I think I went 3:30pm there for the leavers fair and everybody was saying, 'Jasmeen, you made nice, wonderful bhel, we love it.' I think it's finished within half an hour. The school they like it.

In summary then, Jasmeen's lunchbox can be described as confidently Indian with some innovative variations to combine food practices from Britain and to cater for her daughter's preferences. Home food and lunchbox food appear to fit together without any issues within her narrative.

Danijela's chorizo sandwiches

Danijela lives in London in a shared ownership (part buy/ part rent) house and is originally from Croatia. She is married and works full time in a professional and scientific occupation, while her husband is Spanish and works in the transport industry. They have two children aged 8 and 10. Danijela explained that both she and her husband like to cook but it is more practical for her to do it due to working hours.

Both children tried school dinners but then asked to change to packed lunches. Danijela described the typical composition of her children's lunchboxes:

> Well, [my daughter] will have pasta. Yes, so basically, [my son] will not have the pasta. So she will the pasta. Then, they both have either a tortilla or a sandwich, with either ham, chorizo, cheese, sometimes meatballs, sometimes if we have leftover chicken with mayonnaise. Then, they will have a yogurt, an apple, and they will have Belvita, I think it is called, or they will have a packet of popcorn, or they will sometimes have a Cheestring. So it depends what we buy for the week, yes.
>
> Well, we all like tortilla, so tortilla is something that he [her son] really likes, so I know that he is going to eat it. Again, ham, I know he is going to eat ham and cheese. Chorizo is what she is eating. I tried him with pasta and he would not try it. So he would basically come back with a full pot. So I stopped doing that.

Danijela's approach to lunchboxes is infused with influences from Spanish food. In describing her children's lunchboxes, she explained that her son was particularly fussy and neither child would eat vegetables in their lunchbox. Possibly as a result of this, Danijela also expressed negative feelings towards lunchboxes as unhealthy.

INTERVIEWER: How do you feel about making them?
DANIJELA: I hate them.
INTERVIEWER: Oh, why is that?
DANIJELA: I hate them. I hate it because I just think it is not very healthy. Mainly it is sandwiches and these little things. I think it is just really bad basically.
INTERVIEWER: You continue giving them …
DANIJELA: Packed lunches.
INTERVIEWER: Because the children ask or for another reason?
DANIJELA: Because otherwise, he will not eat at school, so …
INTERVIEWER: So it is better that he has that then?
DANIJELA: At least something, yes. Then, I make sure that in the evening, they have proper meals, yes.

Danijela does not only see lunchboxes as 'bad' because of the processed content which she highlighted, but also because she also sees them as culturally different and, in her words, 'very English'. She explained that:

Because I grew up in Croatia and for us, the main meal is lunch so we always had a really healthy lunch. We would be in school until lunchtime and we would go home to eat lunch. So for me, to have a sandwich for lunch is just really weird. I would have a sandwich for dinner, but for lunch, I just find it is really weird. I am kind of getting used to all this and obviously I am doing it, so, yes.

Having to feed her 'picky son' who will not eat the food provided by the school, Danijela sees lunchboxes as a cultural imposition on her way of mothering, since she gives her son some food she considers to be unhealthy. She explained that: 'I just think a sandwich is just a bad thing to have five times a week … Because it is bread, and processed cheese, and processed meat. Yes, I do not like it.'

For Danijela there appears to be a disconnection between food provided at home and in the packed lunch. Unlike Jasmeen, Danijela's lunchboxes do not provide a connection to her childhood. Yet she continues to provide them for her children, and to fit this domestic labour into the morning before she goes to work. Despite 'hating them', they are framed as the only way of doing mothering and putting her child's needs and preferences first. Worried about her son being hungry for long periods, she prioritises food that her son will eat. As such, she accommodates his requests, which symbolises how her mothering is perceived to be compromised by what she considers to be a bad food culture.

Luiz's fajita

Originally from Latin America, Luiz has lived in Canada and Europe before coming to the UK. His wife is from Canada and both he and his wife are working in demanding professional roles. They own their own home in an affluent area in Surrey. Employed full time in the finance industry but undertaking relatively flexible hours from home or commuting into work in London later in the day, he is involved with the childcare of his two daughters, aged 4 and 9.

Variety of food, including varieties of dishes, is considered very important for the children's and the family's diet. This is reflected by their means of acquiring food, which is a weekly delivery of organic vegetables:

> We actually get a lot of our food delivered by Abel & Cole. So the bulk of our produce is Abel & Cole, and we supplement that with trips to Sainsbury's. Partly convenience of delivery, although supermarkets also deliver. But the real driving force was their organic produce and the fact that it's locally sourced. My wife is very keen on that. Also the variety. When you go to the supermarket you can become stuck in a rut; you always buy the same things. Abel & Cole once a week provide you with some very odd vegetable or fruit.

Luiz explained that the use of these vegetable boxes inspires them to try out new dishes as there may be foods in there that they are not familiar with. Such food may form part of a dish within the packed lunches. Luiz explained that his lunchboxes always include fresh fruit and vegetables. Referring to his eldest daughter, Luiz explained that:

> She sometimes takes a sandwich, but more often than not we send her with a hot meal in a thermos flask – a white thermos flask. That can be something left over from the night before or it's something that we prepare in the morning or heat up in the morning.

Thermos flasks were a popular development among the middle-class respondents in the sample at the time of the research (Harman and Cappellini, 2015). Luiz contrasts the lunchboxes he and his wife prepare for their daughters with the packed lunches he consumed during his own childhood (sandwiches with processed white bread) and he argues that the increased understanding of healthy eating, which began before he had his children, has been very important. Although not explicitly criticizing his own upbringing, the lunchboxes his daughters receive are positioned as 'better' and 'healthier'.

Echoing the middle-classes' ideals of what a good diet should be (Wills et al., 2011), Luiz explains that heath, self-discipline as well as a broader repertoire of dishes are the main pillars of the family food. It is in this variety of food experiences offered to the children that fajitas are included. If Jasmeen's chapati was described as a sign her cultural heritage, for Luiz including fajitas, fresh guacamole and other examples of 'food from the world' in his children's lunchboxes seems to be positioned as part of a cosmopolitan diet of a middle-class family. It also solves needs relating to healthy eating and time pressures of dual-income families (O'Connell and Brannen, 2016), as food leftover from the previous evening's meals can be repackaged as lunchtime food when working commitments are heightened. Migration and ethnicity here appears to be less salient than social class, and gender is also part of the picture. Preparing lunchboxes is part of the 'help' (his own term) that he provides with domestic work and childcare.

LUIZ: I think my doing them every morning is the simplest thing. I know Hannah does find them stressful and she is grateful ...
INTERVIEWER: Why do you think that is?
LUIZ: I don't really know. I think I'm more methodical than she is. So for me, when I do the lunch boxes, there is this formula and I just follow it from beginning to end. I think perhaps maybe she over thinks it, I don't know. Or she just feels pressured in the morning. Whereas I'm quite happy to just get on with it. She does express appreciation for that, so I can't lose, can I? Lunches get done and I get appreciated. Having said that, I will start and do the main part of the lunch box and I might ask her to just put the fruit in and she's happy to do that. So long as I've done the bulk of it, then it eases the morning. I don't find it a big deal, so that works out fine.

This extract suggests that Luiz is partly motivated in his endeavour to provide lunchboxes by smoothing relations with his wife and receiving appreciation. Using his terms, he was happy to *'help her out'*, which implies that feeding the family was still seen primarily as her responsibility (see Molander, this volume). Interestingly, appreciation from a spouse was not a reason cited for preparing lunchboxes by any of female respondents. Instead, mothers' narratives most commonly invoked concerns around control over children's diets and the desire to make sure children's needs were being met.

For Luiz and his family, there appears to be a fluid relationship between food consumed at home and taken to school in the lunchbox. Within his lunchbox preparation process, cultural meanings related to good middle-class parenting, healthy eating and being an involved father are visible.

Discussion

The three brief stories of Jasmeen, Danijela and Luiz have highlighted some of the ideals, ideas, emotions and understandings inside children's lunchboxes. As Metcalfe and colleagues (2008) remind us, such understandings are culturally embedded, and as such lunchboxes are balanced culturally rather than nutritionally. Like every other meal, food served in lunchboxes reflects a wider structure and a cosmology (Douglas 1972) of familial bonds and relationship, gender and power structure within the family and conviviality in the private and public sphere. Perhaps learning to balance lunchboxes culturally is more complex than any other meals, since they are prepared in the home but displayed and scrutinised in public settings, in which moralising questions about good parenting, cultural identity and Britishness might be raised.

The three examples show different ways of responding to packed lunches. Jasmeen sees lunchboxes as an opportunity to maintain her own culture, perpetuating ideas and practices of mothering that she learnt from her own mother and communicating her and her daughter's identity within the school context. As Indian food is part of the British culture and marketplace, she does not encounter obstacles in serving her daughters with dishes that resonates with what can be found in many high streets in Britain. Ingredients are easily available and Indian dishes are celebrated as symbols of a super-diverse country (Vertovec, 2007). It would be useful to do ethnographic research in schools to see if the reception of such food is as welcoming as the commercial discourse. At face value, Jasmeen appears to be in a more favourable position than Danijela, whose lunches she enjoyed as a child seem culturally distant from what she now provides for her children. This speaks to the emotional side of food work (Chowbey, 2017). Framed as a cultural imposition, her lunchboxes materialise a resentment towards a culture, and maybe a cosmology to echo Douglas (1972), that is alien to Danijela's ideas of good parenting and good food. As Croatian culinary culture does not have a prominent presence in the current British food culture and marketplace, Danijela might have found it more difficult to reproduce food from 'home' in her children's lunchboxes. Drawing on culinary influences from Spain appears to offer Daniela some opportunities to incorporate the cooked food she values into her children's lunchboxes, but she remains concerned about the processed content and the lack of fresh vegetables (which she explains are omitted because they will not be eaten). A different perspective is then offered by Luiz, whose fajitas are not presented as part of his cultural heritage, but as 'food from the world', and inserted in a typical middle-class narrative of privileged access to a varied, healthy, broad and adventurous diet. As Luiz's narrative is aligned with the normative discourses of parenthood typical of the British middle-class, his lunchboxes are a testimony of integration and working towards a more equal distribution of domestic labour in the household.

The findings suggest the variable salience as ethnicity as a social identity within migrant parents' narratives. For some, ethnicity is explicit, as in Jasmeen's desire to provide the type of lunchtime food she had eaten as a child in India to her own daughter living in London. For others ethnicity initially appeared less salient, but was perhaps significant 'behind the scenes' in contributing to parents' dispositions towards lunch boxes. For example, does Danijela hate lunchboxes because she sees them as culturally alien? Is she hurt by her son's preference for these over food that was more typical in her own childhood, or unhappy about the structure of working life in Britain that does not make returning home for lunch possible? For other parents, ethnicity is present, but overtaken by other social identities such as gender and social class. Being a father who is actively involved in food work, Luiz' narrative stands out as different from other participants and this, combined with the family's middle-class status seem more salient than ethnicity.

The cultural reception of lunchboxes in the school (including reactions from children's peers and school teachers) was not discussed in detail within the interviews and would be an interesting area for future work. The material in this chapter also raises key questions about how far schools and nursery providers foster cultural inclusion by facilitating and valuing a range of food to be brought in for children (Albon, this volume). For future studies, including children's as well as parents' perspectives would increase our understanding of how food gets selected for inclusion in packed lunches, what gets eaten, and how different types of lunchboxes (including those reflecting a range of cultural and ethnic backgrounds) are received in the school setting.

Conclusion

The material discussed within this chapter has suggested that intersectionality is a useful concept when examining parents' perspectives on lunchtime food. It allows us to think about the combination of different influences and the ways in which some may be more important than others within a particular social context. It is not that social class 'trumps' ethnicity, for example, but there is a complicated interface of axes of inclusion and exclusion, markers of similarities and difference within a given time and space. Indeed, intersectionality shows how advantages and disadvantages linked to gender, social class, cultural proximity and inclusion or exclusion to the marketplace, are all at play and visible in the making of children's lunchboxes. Given that food continues to be an important vehicle for expressing and passing on social identities, this remains an important area for social research.

References

Alibhai-Brown, Y. (2009) *The Settlers Cookbook: A Memoir of Love, Migration and Food*, Granta.
Allison, A. (1991) Japanese mothers and obentos: the lunch-box as ideological state apparatus, *Anthropological Quarterly*, 64(4), pp. 195–208.
Barn, R.Ladino, C. and Rogers, C. (2006) *Parenting in Multi-Racial Britain*. London: NCB.
Becher, H. (2008) *Family Practices in South Asian Muslim Families*. Basingstoke: Palgrave.
Cappellini, B. and D.A. Yen (2016) A space on one's own: spatial and identity liminality in an online community of mothers, *Journal of Marketing Management*, 32(13–14), pp. 1260–1283.

Cappellini, B. Harman, V. and Parsons, E. 'Unpacking the Lunchbox: Biopedagogies, Mothering and Social Class' *Sociology of Health and Illness*. https://doi.org/10.1111/1467-9566.12751 (advanced access published online 19. 06. 18).

Chowbey, P. (2017) What is food without love? The micro-politics of food practices among South Asians in Britain, India, and Pakistan, *Sociological Research Online*, 22(3).

Crenshaw, K. (1989) Demarginalizing the intersection of race and sex: a black feminist critique of antidiscrimination doctrine, feminist theory and antiracist politics, *University of Chicago Legal Forum*, pp. 138–167.

Daniel, P. and Gustafsson, U. (2010) School lunches: children's services or children's spaces? *Children's Geographies*, 8(3), pp. 265–274.

DeVault, M. (1991) *Feeding the Family: The Social Organisation of Caring as Gendered Work*. Chicago, IL: University of Chicago Press.

Donner, H. (2006) Committed mothers and well-adjusted children: privatisation, early-years education and motherhood in Calcutta, *Modern Asian Studies*, 40(2), pp. 371–395.

Douglas, M. (1972) Deciphering a meal, *Daedalus*, 101(1), pp. 61–81.

Fathi, M. (2017) *Intersectionality, Class and Migration: Narratives of Iranian Women Migrants in the UK*. New York: Palgrave.

Garner, S. (2010) *Racisms: An Introduction*. London: Sage.

The Guardian (19. 04. 01) *Robin Cook's chicken tikka masala speech* www.theguardian.com/world/2001/apr/19/race.britishidentity (last accessed 17. 12. 17).

Harman, V. and Cappellini, B. (2014), Unpacking fun food and children's leisure: mothers' perspective on preparing lunchboxes, *Young Consumers*, 15(4), pp. 312–322.

Harman, V. and Cappellini, B. (2015) Mothers on display: lunchboxes. Social class and moral accountability, *Sociology*, 49(4), pp. 764–781.

Harman, V. and Cappellini, B. (2017) Boxed up? Lunchboxes and expansive mothering outside home, *Families, Relationships and Societies*. www.ingentaconnect.com/content/tpp/frs/pre-prints/content-ppfrsd1600035r3 (Advanced access published online 14. 08. 17).

Hodges, C.E.M. and Wiggins, G. (2013) Three families—one street: a study of culture, food, and consumption in East London, *Family and Consumer Sciences Research Journal*, 41, pp. 254–266.

Hollows, J. and Jones, S. (2010) "At least he's doing something": moral entrepreneurship and individual responsibility in Jamie's Ministry of Food, *European Journal of Cultural Studies*, 13(3), pp. 307–322.

hooks, bell (1981) *Ain't I a Woman*. Boston, MA: South End Press.

Karrebæk, S.M. (2012) "What's in your lunch box today?": health, respectability, and ethnicity in the primary classroom, *Journal of Linguistic Anthropology*, 22(1), pp. 1–22.

Metcalfe, A., Owen, J., Shipton, G. and Dryden, C. (2008) Inside and outside the school lunchbox: themes and reflections, *Children's Geographies*, 6(4), pp. 403–412.

O'Connell, R. and Brannen, J. (2016) *Food, Families and Work*, London: Bloomsbury Academic.

Oswald, L.R. (1999) Culture swapping: consumption and the ethnogenesis of middle-class Haitian immigrants, *Journal of Consumer Research*, 25(March), pp. 303–318.

Pike, J. (2008) Foucault, space and primary school dining rooms, *Children's Geographies*, 6(4), pp. 413–422.

Pike, J. and Leahy, D. (2012) School food and the pedagogies of parenting, *Australian Journal of Adult Learning*, 52(3), pp. 434–459.

Pitcher, R. (2014) *Consuming Race*, London: Routledge.

Roberts, M. and Pettigrew, S. (2013) Psychosocial influences on children's food consumption, *Psychology and Marketing*, 30(2), pp. 103–120.

Sekhon, Y.K. (2007) "From saris to sarongs": ethnicity and intergenerational influences on consumption among Asian Indians in the UK, *International Journal of Consumer Studies*, 31, pp. 160–167.

Skeggs, B. (2004) *Class, Self, Culture*, London: Routledge.

Venkatesh, A. (1995) Ethnoconsumerism: A New Paradigm to Study Cultural and Cross-cultural Consumer Behavior, in J.A. Costa & G. Bamossy (eds.), *Marketing in a Multicultural World*, Thousand Oaks, CA: SAGE Publications. pp. 26–67.

Vertovec, S. (2007) Super-diversity and its implications, *Ethnic and Racial Studies*, 30(6) pp. 1024–1054.

Vincent, C., Rollock, N., Ball, S. and Gillborn, D. (2012) Intersectional work and precarious positionings: Black middle class parents and their encounters with schools in England, *International Studies in Sociology of Education*, 22(3) pp. 259–276.

Wills, W., Backett-Milburn, K., Roberts, M. and Lawton, J. (2011) The framing of social class distinctions through family food and eating practices, *The Sociological Review*, 59(4) pp. 725–740.

Yuval-Davis, N. (2006) Intersectionality and feminist politics, *European Journal of Women's Studies*, 13(3) pp. 193–209.

Chapter 4

School meal reform and feeding ordering in Portugal
Conventions and controversies

Mónica Truninger and Rosa Sousa

Introduction

Children and young people's food practices are nowadays more visible, surveyed and contested than ever before. There are unprecedented levels of public and media discussion concerning young people's practices, their exposure to marketing and advertisements, concerns around their health, education, leisure activities, internet safety, and eating. Regarding the latter, food issues have gained increasing attention from the media and conquered central stage in the policy agendas of several countries. For example, in the UK, the growing interest in children and food consumption is visible in several policy initiatives that commenced in the present century (see Graham et al., this volume). Some of these attempted to tackle the perceived unbalanced nutritional quality of school meals, to encourage children to eat better (e.g. reduced intake of sugary, fatty foods and fizzy drinks). Other than the UK, more countries are putting considerable efforts to reform school meals towards healthier and nutritionally balanced meals including sourcing organic and local produce, thus combining an agenda of health with one of sustainability (Morgan and Sonnino, 2008).

Portugal carried out a school meal reform after years of relative disinterest that characterized most of the 1990s. In 2006, new standards and guidelines for school meals were launched to tackle rising levels of excess weight and obesity among children, a problem that was worrying health experts at the time[1]. Thus, children's eating practices have been perceived as 'risky' and 'problematic' for their bodies and health states (James, Kjorholt and Tingstad, 2009). Despite the media-influenced public and political visibility of children's food consumption in Portugal, there is scant attention on the principles and values that inform such school meal reform (conducive to a particular way of engaging with school meals, and ultimately, food tastes) and on the effects produced by it on the organization of school meals and children's food practices. Such effects triggered controversy, tensions and mismatches between school meals principles and practices (Truninger, Horta and Teixeira, 2014).

Informed by theoretical approaches that contribute to a 'pragmatic turn' in social sciences, which are more 'attentive to the dynamics of action' (Thévenot, 2007, p. 410) this chapter focuses on two controversies – school meal organization and children's tastes – and identifies the conventions put forward by different actors. It also looks at the ways such controversies were acquiesced through provisional compromises. The empirical material is drawn from focus groups with children, interviews with teachers, kitchen staff and local authorities, and direct observation of lunch meals in the canteens of two nursery/primary schools sited in Lisbon Metropolitan Area at two different periods in time – 2011/2012 and 2015/2016 – that is, during and after the peak of the economic crisis.

The chapter is organized in five sections. First, we review the literature on school meals and children's eating practices before conceptually exploring the notion of 'feeding ordering'. We draw on the work of Law (1994) and Boltanski and Thévenot (1991) to guide this conceptual exploration. Second, we explain the methodological procedures and describe the empirical material collected. Third, we analyse the national school meal reform over the last ten years, informed by the above conceptual framework. Fourth, we examine a case study of two schools in the municipality of Cascais and seek to understand the conventions underlying the justifications to set up a series of changes in the school food provisioning system, which gave rise to a particular feeding ordering underpinned by a bundle of conventions. We also look at the way actors of the school meals system dealt with two controversies – the school meals organization and children's tastes – and how they managed to adjust their practices and principles to suspend such controversies by making compromises. The final section provides a summary of the findings and a critical reflection on the heuristic value of employing a pragmatic sociological approach in order to analyse school meals.

School meals reform and main controversies

Schools have been identified as an important site for intervention in relation to children's eating habits. Several schools worldwide have set up school meal reforms with the hope of solving perceived problems with the health status of children. These interventions and policy measures tend to frame children's eating habits as problematic and risk-related (James, Kjorholt, Tingstad, 2009). In this policy context, eating is often defined as a medical problem, to be solved with the provision of the 'right balance' of calorie intake and output (Pike 2008; Gustafsson, 2004). Looking at Portuguese schools meals, Truninger et al. (2013) showed that there is an increasing effort by policymakers to engage (on paper) in a more holistic view of health, going beyond food as nutrition. However, in practice a biomedical understanding of school meals still pervades in the spaces where children eat. Children associate food in the canteen with nutrition and health, whereas food associated with 'pleasure' is found in the competing retail food shops that surround the schools. Other studies found similar ways of classifying food by children in binary categories, with healthy food associated with the 'home' and 'junk' food associated with pleasure, friends and weight gain (Ludvigsen and Scott, 2009: 421).

Since the beginning of the 21st century calls for improving food in schools have been especially copious, often identifying childhood rates of obesity and excessive weight as the 'hook' for action and intervention (Best, 2017). However, changing school meals affects more than nutritional intake, touching upon the multidimensional character of food (Morgan, 2014). As stated by Andersen (2015: 3), 'the strict focus on risk and nutrition overlooks the cultural meanings that food bears, as well as the social processes that surround children's eating practices', that is, the relationships children establish with their carers and peers in school (Truninger and Teixeira, 2015). School meals are also seen as an opportunity for food education given their capacity to teach children about food, nutrition, meal norms and rules through practice, by experimenting in the canteen unfamiliar tastes and flavours (Andersen, 2015; Morgan & Sonnino 2008). However, the disciplining and nutritional features of school meals give rise to controversies when implementing such changes (see Albon, this volume). Research has found that staff has often an authoritarian approach regarding children's eating practices in schools, to retain control over children (Morrison, 1996; Pike, 2008; Dotson, Vaquera and Cunningham, 2015). Teaching staff tend to check if children bring healthy or junk food to school and judge these practices irrespective of the socioeconomic or cultural context of the family (Leahy, 2010). Daniel and Gustafsson (2010) found several processes of tension between institutional constraints (school meals as 'children's services') and children food practices in the canteen while getting served, eating and going out to play (school meals as 'children's spaces'). In this case, there was a cleavage between adult-children roles and expectations towards eating school meals. There is already a solid body of work showing the strategies of resistance by children to eating school meals (Dotson, Vaquera and Cunningham, 2015; Truninger and Teixeira, 2015) and the importance of children's peers in accepting or rejecting the food on offer in schools (Andersen et al, 2016). However, it is relevant to consider the social, material and moral embeddedness of school meals, and how children and staff experience and appropriate the norms and rules set up by policies on school meals. In this chapter, we will look at some of the controversies created by the implementation of a school meal reform in Portugal. We will examine how these controversies are rooted in a multiplicity of dimensions that go beyond health and nutrition. To help in the conceptualization of a passage from a monolithic understanding of school meals (based on biomedical and nutritional features) to a plural and multiple understanding of school meals we explore the potential of combining conventions theory and Law's concept of ordering.

Conventions theory develops in the mid-1980s from the works of French authors such as Luc Boltanski, Laurent Thévenot, Robert Salais, Jean Pierre Dupuy, François Eymard-Duvernay, Olivier Favereau, and André Orléan. Conventions are understood as 'modes of evaluation' used by individuals to interpret action in specific and situated contexts (Ponte and Gibbon, 2005). In ambiguous situations such as the ones provoked by a controversy actors resource to particular moral evaluations (underpinned by a limited plurality of 'orders of worth') and objects (materials, artefacts) in order to cease the controversy and coordinate action with others. Thus, both human and nonhuman, people and objects, articulate and configure the so-called 'pragmatic regimes' (Thévenot, 2001b) in which two components are included: one is the moral component that shapes the legitimate principles of evaluation employed by the actors in a particular situation; the other is the involvement of objects or 'material reality' employed as 'proof' of the arguments at stake. The regime of justification encompasses criticism and disputes where arguments are framed by the highest degree of legitimacy – conventions. These are incorporated into different 'orders of worth'. Each 'order of worth' is based on common superior principles of qualification (or "common good"), which are forms of collective evaluation used in the processes of criticism, denunciation and compromise (Thévenot, 2001a). Thus, in everyday life different actors engage in disparate situations that lead them to use bundles of conventions to justify their practices, their views, or even their reasons to implement, for example, a school meal reform (Table 4.1).

The list of orders of worth on Table 4.1 is the original one proposed by Boltanski and Thévenot's early works. The authors suggested six moral orders as they can usually be found in claims and justifications of many situations in the contemporary French context. This is not a closed list and more orders can be added (e.g. the green order), but for the sake of the controversies on school meals in the Portuguese context, these six orders are sufficient to interpret the ways in which different actors engage in disputes for the quality of school meals. Each of these 'orders of worth' exists in a state of tension, because they try to resist or encroach into other "orders" (Raikes, Jensen and Ponte, 2000: 408). For example, in this claim 'school meals should be healthier, they use very cheap foods' there is a denunciation of the quality of school meals because of its price (market conventions are criticised). On the other hand, it displays the principle from which this denunciation is made (civic conventions are valued, namely the health principle that should be universal, supporting the common good of public health). Sometimes these controversies are resolved, and the government re-allocates some of its budget to provide better and healthier meals in schools. For example, the instance when Tony Blair's government decided to invest more funding into school food in the wake of Jamie Oliver's 'School

Table 4.1 Moral orders and school meals controversies

Orders of worth	Main Principle	Mode of evaluation	Controversy
Market	Competition	Price	The cost of the school meal service is too high
Industrial	Efficiency	Productivity, technical efficiency, measurable criteria	The technical procedures for school meals (size of portions, food safety norms) are too cumbersome
Civic	Collective	Equality, solidarity, collective interest (health, environment, social justice)	School meals are unhealthy. School meals are not environmentally friendly
Domestic	Tradition	Trustworthiness, familiar ties, esteem	School meals are not home-cooked food
Inspired	Inspiration	Aesthetics, flavour, taste of the meal, pleasure, emotions	School meals are tasteless, they look bland and unappetising
Opinion	Public opinion	Recognition, popularity, media	School meals are not prepared by celebrity chefs

Source: Adapted on the basis of Boltanski and Thévenot (1999: 368) and Andersen (2011: 443).

Dinners' Campaign in the UK (Pike and Kelly, 2014). Thus, compromises are established and agreed between different orders of worth. As put by Boltanski and Thévenot (1999: 374): 'In a compromise, people maintain an intentional proclivity towards the common good by cooperating to keep present beings relevant in different worlds, without trying to clarify the principle upon which their agreement is grounded'. In the example above we have a school meal policy that is composed of both market and civic conventions, where price and health are combined to offer a quality meal. It is this idea of composition that is important to link with Law's conceptual framework. We engage here with his concept of order*ing*, given its open-ended, provisional, messy and heterogeneously composite status. As argued by Law (1994: 1–2) 'orders are never complete. Instead they are more or less precarious and partial accomplishments that may be overturned. They are, in short, better seen as verbs than nouns'. This is why order*ing* (as a verb) is more appropriate to capture the plural, incompleteness and messy processes of the world, and in our case, the evolving processes of setting up changes in the school meals system in Portugal. Moreover, as explained by Law, ordering is composed of heterogeneous elements, be they human or non-human. Thus, talk, bodies, texts, technologies, canteen layouts, tables dispositions and foods are implicated in a particular 'feeding ordering'. Linking the two bodies of work, we suggest that feeding ordering is the outcome and effect of plural ordering modes. These ordering modes encapsulate orders of worth governed by market, domestic, industrial, opinion, inspiration or civic conventions. The advantage of this analytical exploration is to qualify Law's concept of ordering with these different conventions, and to stress the incompleteness, messiness and precarious organization that the concept order*ing* offers to an informed convention theory analysis of school meals' justifications, controversies and compromises. Both 'order*ing*' and 'conventions' can be inscribed in a 'pragmatic turn', and both are theoretically situated in post-structuralist approaches where humans and non-humans are treated symmetrically. They also decentre the analytic perspective from a single/individual order (e.g. nutrition/health) to 'multiple modes of order*ing*', in Law's language, or, if we take Boltanski and Thévenot's lingo, to a 'limited plurality of orders of worth' (e.g. market, domestic, industrial).

Methodological procedures

The empirical material used in this chapter is drawn from two different research projects. The first entailed a three-year project entitled 'Between School and Family: Children's Food Knowledge and Eating Practices', which was carried out during the peak of the economic crisis that severely affected Portugal (2011–2014). The main aim of this project was to look at the school meal reform of 2006 and describe the effects of such reform on the organization of school meals, children's eating practices, and parents' views of family and food. We conducted 18 focus groups in eight primary and secondary schools across the country with both children (from 8–10 and 11–14 years old) and parents, together with interviews with the teachers, the catering companies, local authorities and the kitchen staff. We also conducted direct observation in canteens, school playgrounds and the school's surrounding shops. For this chapter, we use only a small portion of the material collected, namely a focus group with 10 primary school children aged between 8 and 10 years old, an interview with the city council and five interviews with the kitchen and teaching staff of a primary school located in the municipality of Cascais (Lisbon Metropolitan Area).

The second project is part of a PhD in its final stages entitled 'Public Procurement and Sustainable Development: The Case of Schools', wherein the fieldwork covers the period after the peak of the crisis, i.e., 2015/2016. This project aims to analyse public procurement initiatives, which combine health and sustainability to ensure that school meals are nutritiously balanced, source local and organic foods when possible, and reduce food waste. The data used for this chapter refers to interviews conducted with the kitchen and teaching staff from a nursery school of Cascais, the catering company that supplies the food to the school and two representatives of the city council that oversee the school catering system (totalling 5 interviews). Direct observation of the lunches in the canteens during three school visits were also conducted. The methodological procedures were validated by the Ministry of Education, whereas the permissions for interviews, observation in the canteens, and use of visual methods (photos, videos) were granted by the directors of the schools, the parents and children through informed consent forms. The interviews were fully transcribed and analysed using NVivo 10, together with photos and video recordings. The analysis of the material followed the procedures of a thematic analysis where data were coded and the main patterns were sought considering an iterative process with the theoretical insights convoked to this analysis.

A case study of two primary schools in Cascais

The case study under analysis is situated in Cascais, a town that is sited nearby Lisbon in Portugal. In 2015, the municipality of Cascais (composed of four parishes) had 209,869 inhabitants, of which 16% were children and young people below 15 years old (PORDATA, 2017). Almost 10% of its population were immigrants. About 7.2% were unemployed, 2.2% receives the social integration income, and 2.3% were granted the unemployment allowance. In this council there were 84 state funded primary schools.

The first primary school that we contacted in 2011 is situated in a small parish of Cascais. This primary school (which includes a nursey school as well) is attended by children aged between 6 and 9 years old enrolled in the 1st to 4th grade. In the school year of 2011/2012 there were 180 students overall (15 in the nursery school). The population is of low ethnic diversity, composed of some families of average socio-economic levels, and mainly individuals with low income and poor schooling levels who have been affected by the growing unemployment rates, due to the economic crisis that affected the country between 2008 and 2014.

The second school was approached in the school year 2015/2016 and is sited on the same council but located in a different parish than the previous school. It is a nursery school with 40 children at that time. The education cycle covers children from 3 to 6 years of age. Pre-school education is inserted in a larger school grouping of primary and secondary schools. The headquarters of the grouping – a primary school – was also visited, given that the school meals for the nursery were prepared in its large central kitchen, which also supplied meals to three other schools. The nursery catchment area is characterized by a well-off white population with middle to high levels of education and low unemployment levels. In 2015, economic growth was picking up nationally which contrasted with the previous period of greater hardship among some families living in the council.

The space surrounding both schools features several commercial establishments (coffee shops, supermarkets), some of which specifically target the student population, selling them cheap excess fat and sugary meals that compete with the food served in the canteen. In both schools, most children eat lunch at the canteen and there are strong restrictions against leaving the school during the day. School teachers often monitor the snacks and other foods children bring from home. The council manages the school food provision through a contract with a national food catering company. This company has been supplying the council's schools for more than 13 years. It prepares and cooks the meals directly in the school kitchens (when they are equipped with one) or cooks the meals in three primary school kitchens and then delivers them to the schools without in house catering services. The meals are then brought by van to these schools (the case for our nursery school). As we will see below, the way food is prepared and cooked is a bone of contention regarding children's school meals acceptance.

The school meals reform in Portugal: a brief overview

In 2006, Portugal's National Programme for Healthy Schools (Ministry of Health, 2006) was designed and launched to encourage initiatives that tackle childhood obesity. The objective of this programme was to develop schools' role and responsibility in improving food provision, to ensure that children had access to a nutritionally balanced meal with reduced fat, sugar and salt contents. In the school year 2005/2006, the Generalized Provision of School Meals Programme for Primary School Children was implemented. The programme aimed to encourage all councils of the country to take full accountability for the school meals management and provision (until then only a few councils were taking such responsibilities by fully or partially subsidizing the meals of low income families), and to ensure that all children with extracurricular activities in school could have a midday hot meal. This encouraged the councils to organize a systematic and uninterrupted food catering service, and many outsourced the school meals to private companies. One impact of this measure was the rise in the number of students using the school canteen, when before they would go home to have lunch[2]. Some councils invested a portion of their budgets in activating previously decommissioned school kitchens or equipping new schools with good working kitchens. As we will see, this was an action followed by the Cascais council.

In 2007, school meals' guidelines were launched to guide catering and kitchen staff to prepare the meals according to capitations appropriate to the different children's ages. The menu was composed of three courses with a set of recommendations for nutritionally balanced meals: the starter entailed a fresh vegetable soup, the main course featuring one meat or fish/seafood dish offered in alternate days, accompanied by side dishes of pulses, vegetables, pasta, rice or potatoes (deep frying was highly discouraged), brown bread, and a dessert of seasonal fruit made available daily. Only once a week children were offered one of these options: jelly, ice cream, yoghurt, cooked or baked fruit with no added sugar. The only drink allowed was water.

Another important policy was the European Fruit Distribution Regime[3]. It was launched in 2009, soon adapted to the national legal system and implemented in the school year of 2010–2011 through the National Strategy of School Fruit Regime 2010–2013. The implementation of this strategy aimed to increase children's health protection by improving their intake and knowledge of fruits. In 2012 the General Directorate for Health oversaw the implementation of the first National Programme for the Promotion of Healthy Eating (PNPAS) with several objectives, one among them to encourage the adoption of the Mediterranean Diet among the Portuguese population and to support children in schools to eat healthy meals based on those dietary principles[4]. In 2013, more detailed instructions were introduced on authorized foods, meals composition, menu components, the use of aromatic herbs, and the reduction of salt (Truninger et al., 2015: 48). In 2017, a new referral for health education was launched in June with a large section dedicated to food education. A wider and holistic approach to food is visible, encompassing a variety of topics including nutrition, environmental issues, social justice, Mediterranean Diet, shopping and labelling and the right to food among others.

Informed by the concepts of 'conventions' and 'ordering' we can grasp how these policies encapsulated a feeding ordering underpinned by civic conventions where health concerns were prominent. However, the concerns with the meal cost[5], food safety and hygiene technical requirements in food preparation were also visible. Market conventions (meal price) and industrial conventions (technical procedures and efficiency of the service) underlie such principles. This feeding ordering was essentially underpinned by the composition of civic (health), market (price) and industrial (efficiency) conventions. However, as more policies and initiatives were added, other concerns were pushed to the front, with domestic and civic (environment) conventions becoming more visible. For instance, the backing up of traditional and cultural food values, table manners and socializing (all embracing the ideas of commensality that feature in the Mediterranean Diet), and environmental concerns (food waste reduction). However, coordinating action in this composite and provisional feeding ordering according to such a wide bundle of conventions was not a smooth process, and controversies emerged during the implementation of this reform, as analysed in the following sections.

Feeding ordering and controversies: justifications and compromises

We examine two problems that emerged when the council of Cascais consolidated its action in the management of school meals from 2005/2006 onwards. One problem concerned the process of the meal's preparation and cooking that had to be adjusted to avoid complaints by both children and parents. The other problem (still ongoing) regarded the acceptance of some dishes, namely fish-based meals. Children showed resistance to some school meals and several adjustments to the menus and the cooking procedures had to be made to ensure they accepted dishes better. Both problems emerged with the new feeding ordering triggered by the school meal reform. By exploring cross-fertilization between convention theory and Law's concept of 'ordering' we show the convocation of different conventions and the arrangement of compromises to suspend such controversies, that are, notwithstanding, always precarious ordering accomplishments.

From cook-chill, through temperature control to home cooked food in schools

In the school year of 2005/2006, the council of Cascais made considerable changes to their school meals provisioning system. Due to the implementation of the Generalized Provision of School Meals Programme for Primary School Children the council was obliged to provide school meals to all children enrolled in the nurseries and primary schools under its jurisdiction, whereas before it mainly focused its attention on the provision of meals to children of low income families. With such obligation, it completely restructured the service of school meals, investing in equipping and refurbishing previously decommissioned school kitchens. In the schools where the material infrastructure would not allow such refurbishments, the food was delivered in insulated shipping containers. That is, it was prepared and transported in vans from three central kitchens (sited in schools with large kitchens), where care and monitoring was given to maintain the temperature throughout the entire journey. The council outsourced the catering services to a private national company that provided meals not only for schools, but also hospitals. In the first phase, some schools were supplied with cook–chill meals, that is, meals that were prepared in a central kitchen, fast chilled, transported cold to the school, and stored in the fridge of the school pantry room. On the day of service the meals were reheated and served to the children. In the primary school under analysis this system operated for some time, until the council invested in equipping the premises with a local kitchen after several complaints by the school staff, children and parents. When we interviewed the head teacher in 2012, he remembered that time:

> In its first phase, the meals were pre-cooked, it was not like it is now where we have a local kitchen. It was another company that supplied the meals, not the current one. The food was pre-frozen and then reheated here (…) because this kitchen was not working … there were problems with the kitchen structure. When the current company won the bid, the work started in the kitchen and we have now the meals prepared by this company on our own kitchen. Before, we had a lot of complaints by the

children and the parents because the food was not tasty... now the service is much better.
(Head teacher, primary school, July 2012)

Investing in refurbishing school kitchens or equipping new schools with their own kitchens has been a priority of the council from 2005. They justify this strategy on two counts: the food tastes like home cooked food; and it is better aligned with their overall strategy of providing healthy quality meals to children.

> Another important thing in our strategy, which is also something that has been taken on board with the experience of the cook–chill: all new schools have a local kitchen, and this has been increasing ... We know that there is much more pleasure and better taste in eating food that is prepared and cooked as close as possible to the little ones ...
> (Representatives of the Cascais council, November, 2011)

> We had the cook–chill system before. And they all hated the cook-chill. When the council changed administration this new councilman was more understanding regarding the school meals, and we tried to replace this system in some schools with the transport of hot meals. The main problem with the cook–chill system was the taste of food ... and it baffled us and also the teachers that the food came in a sealed bag. To see the food in bags was very odd (...) I remember one time I went there and it was rice and beans. The beans looked like popcorn. The rice was dry. Everything had exploded ... it was not well re-heated (...) there were complaints on a daily basis.
> (Representatives of the Cascais council, February, 2016)

The process of food preparation had strong implications for the council's change in strategy to provide quality healthy meals. To avoid the children's rejection of the meals, they decided to replace the cook–chill system with two alternatives: transporting the food hot and equipping schools with local kitchens. The first option was employed when there were no facilities to cook in the school. In these cases (namely the nursery school under study) the meals were prepared off site and distributed by vans on the day, in thermal containers to keep the temperature stable. In this process, maintaining the temperature and complying with the food hygiene and safety technical norms, comprised in the school meals' regulations, was crucial to the company, to avoid any public health issue (e.g. food poisoning). As explained by the nutritionist and quality control technician of the company that oversaw the meals' supply to 52 schools in Cascais:

> There are several kitchens that make the confection. There is a shuttle that transports hot meals to smaller schools (...) as long as the

temperatures are maintained, as long as we can guarantee a safe meal, it works rather well. Before we had the hot transport, we had the pre-cooked meals that go to the oven and are served. This type of meal does not taste like a home cooked meal. There were many complaints. Since we changed to hot transport or prepared the food directly in local kitchens the complaints diminished drastically. In the hot transport, sometimes it is difficult for the cooks to get the right time of stopping the cooking process ... because the food continues to cook inside the thermal containers ... it is an art to stop the cooking just in time ... Another problem with the temperature is when we have a temperature break during the transport. There is always some equipment that allows the regeneration if there is a temperature break .... but it is something that we want to avoid.
(Quality technician and nutritionist of catering company, 2016)

In this case maintaining a stable temperature was important to achieve food safety and to ensure compliance with technical procedures for transporting hot food. The justifications advanced were clearly underpinned by industrial conventions due to the amount of care invested in maintaining the efficiency of this system. Interestingly, in house catering services were praised for achieving better taste and quality; producing meals with a home-cooked taste. This relates to the second option followed by the council: to invest in building new kitchens to ensure that school meals were prepared on site and on the day of service. This ensured that the time between meal preparation and consumption was as short as possible, improving the taste, flavor, and overall aesthetics of the meal. The company's head-cook working in the primary school kitchen explained that she tended to cook in the school as she usually does at home. Despite having to comply with strict norms and regulations regarding capitations, salt content and meal portions, she made sure that the emotional investment in cooking the meal in the school premises was the same as when she cooks for her family at home. Despite the strict standards and the large amount of meals to prepare in this school (180 meals a day), the cook considers the work she does similar to that she does at home.

We learn very easily [the new norms] because here we cook as if we were at home, isn't it? The food we make here is exactly like I make in my house ... I'm not doing anything different, I do everything the same. And so it's the same, the salads are the same, it's all the same. There are only those things that we do different here ... for example, we have to be careful to always wash our hands ... but the food here is very similar to the one we cook at home.
(Interview with the school cook, June, 2012)

This way, the cook managed to make a compromise between the technical procedures demanded by the school meals' guidelines (underpinned by industrial conventions), and the skills, competences and emotional investment entailed when producing school meals with a taste of home-cooked food (underpinned by domestic conventions). The feeding ordering that emerged with the school meal reform where health, food safety and taste were paramount generated a set of effects that transformed the previous school meal provisioning logistics of Cascais council (e.g. mode of transport, mode of preparing and serving the meals). The former cook–chill school meal provision encountered resistance by children and teachers on taste grounds. With the emergence and enactment of the new feeding ordering, the Cascais council made a series of changes in the logistics of preparing and serving meals (e.g. transporting the food hot and equipping schools with local kitchens). In this emergent feeding ordering constituted by heterogeneous elements of humans and nonhumans (e.g. kitchen staff, new or refurbished local kitchens, cleaning and food safety procedures, thermometers and temperature loggers, and so on) a set of compromises were settled. Notably between the industrial (e.g. food safety) and domestic conventions (school food tasting like home cooked food) making it possible for children to accept school meals. However, it is important to bear in mind that this ordering mode is always contingent and provisional, as we address in the following section.

Children's resistance to school meals and the making of compromises

When we conducted fieldwork in the primary school back in 2011/2012, fish was already an issue in children's tastes. Teachers, kitchen staff, the council's representatives, and the primary school children we interviewed, all agreed: fish is disliked at school. The following is a conversation held in the focus group with children about the likes and dislikes of school meal dishes.

I: What dishes do you like in school?
MARIA: I like everything but sometimes I don't like the soup. I don't like fish either, I just like fish fingers and the pads … meat pads. Sometimes I like the salad when it's seasoned.
I: And you Ana?
ANA: Fish … when the fish comes with bones I don't eat it.
(Focus group with primary school children, 2012)

Children in the focus group complained about fish bones reporting that on fish day they used to eat the sides and leave the fish on the plate. In the group interview, children showed a strong taste for meat. When we returned to Cascais in the school year 2015/2016, the situation remained the same: fish resistance persisted.

In the nursery of Cascais we observed the process of serving the meals and how children engaged with the dish on offer on the day: fish pie. This nursery consists of two classes of 20 children each. Meals are prepared outside the premises in a school relatively close to the one under analysis and are transported hot in vans. When they arrive at the school the catering technicians start serving the contents of the thermal containers on the plates (Figures 4.1 and 4.2). On the day of the visit, in addition to the vegetable soup, the menu consisted of a fish pie, broccoli at the side, and for desert an apple. No soft drinks were allowed in the meals, only water was available at the table, complying with the national school meal policy.

Before the children's arrival at around 11.45am, tables are set with the food contents already served, and are arranged in a circular way, to facilitate chatting around the table. This is one of the strategies to encourage the ideals conveyed by the Mediterranean Diet where commensality and talking around the table is highly valued (Figures 4.3 and 4.4). However, despite the efforts of the staff to ensure a good socializing atmosphere with this spatial arrangement, the meal time is relatively short and synchronized. Children want to eat fast and play, and not spend time around the table (see also Daniel and Gustafsson, 2010).

Because these are children of 6 years-old or less, energy supplies are smaller, so foods such as bread are cut in portions and placed at the centre of the table. During lunch, children eat the food under the teacher's supervision, who assists with cutting the fruit. Some encouragement to eat the meal is offered. That day most children ate school meals because fish was prepared in a way to facilitate acceptance. Fish without bones and shredded in a fish pie is better accepted than a portion of fish on the plate, as explained by the head-cook:

I: What are the foods that children like the least?
HEAD-COOK: It's the fish. Whatever fish it is. Except for fish fingers that we put in the oven. This year we introduced a fish that was no longer served for 3 or 4 years, which is Pollock fillets and they accepted very well ... salmon in salads it also goes well ... we have little food waste on salmon and pollock days. Fish like tuna, or mackerel they also like. But if for example we serve a piece of hake as we had last year then it is difficult ... it is the bones, they have to remove the spine ... we have to shred the fish, like today in a pie, otherwise we have a lot of waste on fish days.
(Interview with the head cook, 2016)

Shredding fish for a pie for example, is one of several adjustments the cooks learned to make during the past years to make sure children eat fish. In this case, a plethora of heterogeneous human and nonhuman elements such as shredded fish without bones (instead of an entire piece of fish with bones), the skills and competences of the cooks to prepare a pie that appeals to

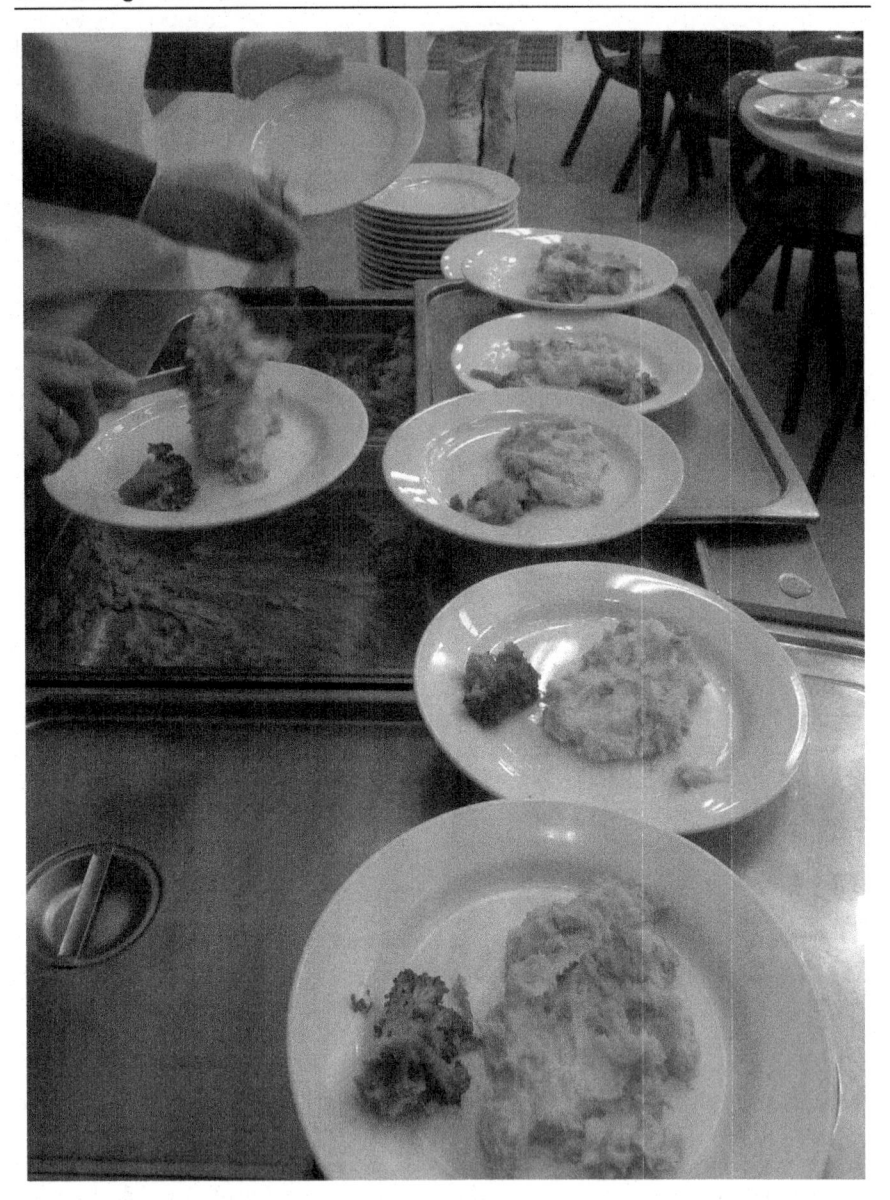

Figure 4.1 Food service in nursery school
Source: Rosa Sousa, 2016.

children's tastes, attentive human eyes to spot and remove the fish bones, and the tools and kitchen equipment for such preparation are all entangled to sustain a mode of ordering where inspiration conventions are encroached. Thus, bringing to the fore the aesthetics of food, such as flavor and texture. However, in this

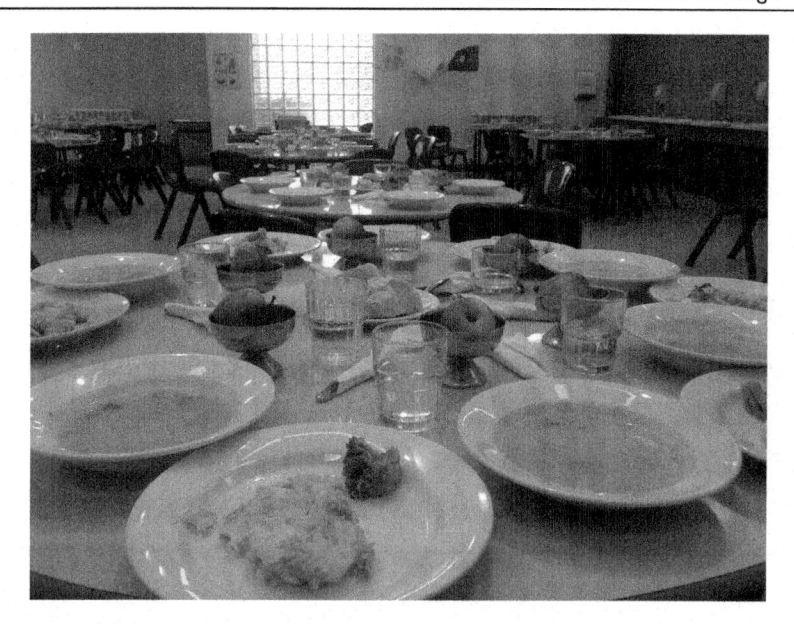

Figure 4.2 Food service in nursery school
Source: Rosa Sousa, 2016.

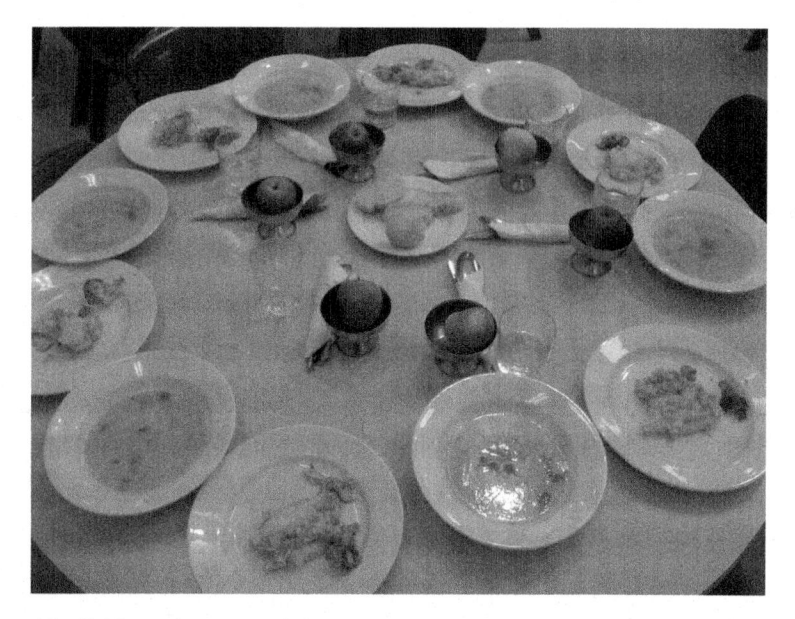

Figure 4.3 Children eating around the table
Source: Rosa Sousa, 2016.

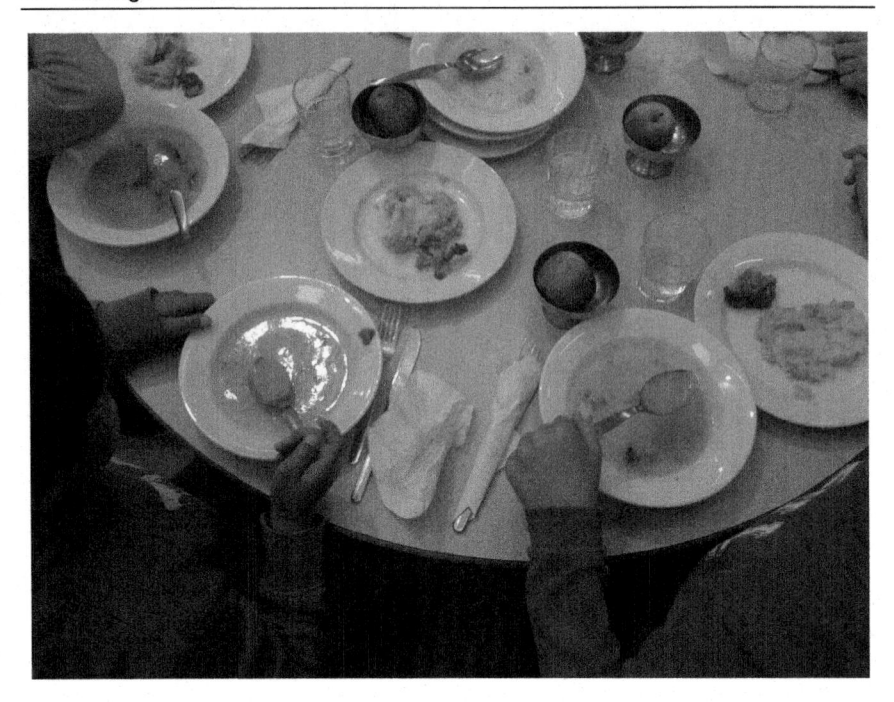

Figure 4.4 Children eating around the table
Source: Rosa Sousa, 2016.

ordering mode aesthetic conventions can also be encroached by civic and market conventions, for example, when food waste is at stake. Both for civic and economic concerns food waste is an issue on fish days. Thus, adjustments to the menus are made (e.g. reducing fish variety) to make sure children eat fish and food is not wasted. Moreover, by reducing fish variety the kitchen staff and the catering company also make compromises between what is written in the contract (which abides by the school meal directives and its technical features) and the daily resistance to fish, its bones and general aesthetics that is felt in the canteen. As explained by the nutritionist of the catering company:

> The menus are based on the school meals norms, but then we need to make some adjustments according to the complaints we received (…). For example, if we have a fish that is in the contract that is not well accepted by the children, we change for another one – like mackerel that they usually like, to make sure they eat fish. The fish variety sometimes is reduced because children struggle to eat all types of fish that we offer … so we tend to give the fish they like. Normally this type of adaptation is almost always in the fish.
> (Quality technician and nutritionist of the catering company, 2016)

In this case, a compromise between industrial conventions (a legal contract with technical procedures) and inspiration conventions (the taste, texture and general aesthetics of the fish as perceived by the children) must be arranged to suspend tension in the canteen. We can observe that inspiration conventions can also be encroached by industrial conventions, both being part of this multiply-constituted mode of ordering. The common good of this mode of ordering revolves around the principle that children need to eat fish due to health reasons (according to the school meals policies), then adjustments and compromises are put in place to ensure civic conventions (health) are enacted. As it was possible to show through our empirical examples, different modes of ordering underpinned by a bundle of conventions (inspiration, health, industrial, market, civic) clashed and adjusted to one another, setting up always precarious and provisional compromises.

Conclusion

This chapter looked at the school meal reform that started in 2005/2006 in Portugal and the composite character of the feeding ordering produced by its new policies. If in the beginning there was a strong focus on a monolithic element of school meals – health concerns were reduced to the nutritional components of food so as to address the risks of childhood obesity and excess weight – a decade later a wider spectrum of values and principles are visible. Thus, several conventions have emerged and circulated over the last 10 years to encourage children to eat in particular ways, and to organize the school meals and the sociotechnical apparatus in the kitchen and canteens according to notions of eating well. These have followed multidisciplinary knowledge and expertise (e.g. nutritional, biomedicine), and have provided foods that convey the principles around safety, hygiene, nutrition, public health, economic saving, food culture, environment, waste, food insecurity among others. However, such proliferation of principles and values would trigger tensions and controversies in the practical implementation of the school meal reform, precisely because school meals are socially, culturally and physically embedded in various ways and cannot be reduced to its nutritional features.

Through qualitative analysis of interviews with teaching, kitchen staff, council's representatives and observations of mealtimes in two schools (one nursery and a primary school) in Cascais, we could examine two controversies. One involved the organization of the school meal through different catering services (cook–chill, insulated shipping containers and in-house catering) and the perception of meal's quality. The other gave an account of children's resistance to fish dishes, and the continuous adjustments made by the cooks to ensure children ate fish. We found that such adjustments are made of compromises between modes of ordering school meals. Such compromises suspend the controversy for a while, but are always precarious and incomplete.

The advantage of pulling together Law's concept of ordering with convention theory was, on the one hand, to stress such incompleteness, messiness and precariousness found in school meals modes of ordering. On the other hand, convention theory offered depth and richness to the qualification of the feeding ordering that emerged from the school meal reform, by unveiling not its monolithic character, but rather its heterogeneity and plurality in the conventions that were mobilized to support different orders of worth.

Acknowledgments

Some of the research leading to these results has received funding from FCT (the Portuguese National Science Agency) through the project 'Between School and Family: Children's Food Knowledge and Eating Practices (PTDC/CS-SOC/111214/2009). We are also grateful for the useful comments offered by an anonymous referee.

Notes

1 Nowadays, this problem continues to be a source of, despite current efforts to tackle childhood excess weight and obesity through several health and education governmental programs. The second national food survey (Lopes et al., 2017) applied in 2015/2016 reports that obesity hits 7.7% of children under 10 years old and 8.7% of adolescents between 10 and 17 years old. Moreover, 68.9% of children and 65.9% of adolescents do not comply with the WHO recommended fruit and vegetables portions per day (400 gr, i.e., 5-a-DAY).
2 According to an evaluation report on the implementation of this programme, in its first year (2005/2006) about 22 million meals were served to primary school children in the whole country. In the year 2011/2012, this number more than doubled reaching over 47 million school meals served nationally (Ministry of Education and Science, 2013).
3 Regulation (CE) n. 288/2009, European Commission.
4 See www.alimentacaosaudavel.dgs.pt/en/pnpas-2/ accessed on 1st March 2017.
5 In the school year 2015/2016 the full price of the meal was €3 per head. However, the price that parents pay is half of this, at €1,50. The Government covers part of this cost while the parents pay the remaining cost. For low income families or families on social benefits free school meals are available, which are fully covered by the State.

References

Andersen, Sidse S. (2015) *School Meals in Children's Social Life: A Study of Contrasting Meal Arrangements*, PhD thesis manuscript, Copenhagen: University of Copenhagen.
Andersen, Sidse S., Ditte Vassard, Louis N. Havn, Camilla T. Damsgaard, Anja Biltoft-Jensen, Lotte Holm (2016) Measuring the impact of classmates on children's liking of school meals, *Food Quality and Preference*, 52, pp. 87–95, ISSN 950–3293, http://dx.doi.org/10.1016/j.foodqual.2016.03.018.
Andersen, Anne H. (2011) Organic food and plural moralities of food provisioning, *Journal of Rural Studies*, 27(4), pp. 440–450.

Best, Amy L. (2017) *Fast-Food Kids: French Fries, Lunch Lines, and Social Ties*, New York: New York University Press.
Boltanski, Luc and Laurent Thévenot (1991) *De la justification. Les economies de grandeur*, Paris: Gallimard.
Boltanski, Luc and Laurent Thévenot (1999) The sociology of critical capacity, *European Journal of Social Theory*, 2(3), p. 359–377.
Boltanski, Luc and Laurent Thévenot (2006) *On justification: Economies of worth*. Translation by Catherine Porter. Princeton, NJ: Princeton University Press.
Daniel, Paul and Ulla Gustafsson (2010) School lunches: children's services or children's spaces? *Children's Geographies*, 8(3), pp. 265–274.
Dotson, Hilary M., Elizabeth Vaquera and Solveig Argeseanu Cunningham (2015) Sandwiches and subversion: teacher's mealtime strategies and preschoolers' agency, *Childhood*, 22(3), pp. 362–376.
Gustafsson, Ulla (2004) The privatisation of risk in school meals policies, *Health, Risk & Society*, 6(1), pp. 53–65.
James, Allison, Anne Trin Kjorholt and Vebjog Tingstad (2009) Introduction: Children, Food and Identity in Everyday life, in Allison James, Anne Trin Kjorholt and Vebjog Tingstad (eds), *Children, Food and Identity in Everyday Life*, Basingstoke: Palgrave, pp. 1–12.
Law, John (1994) *Organizing Modernity*, Oxford: Blackwell.
Leahy, Deana (2010) What's on (or off) the menu in school? *Text. Special Issue: Rewriting the Menu: The Cultural Dynamics of Contemporary Food Choices*, 9, p. 1–12.
Lopes, Carla, Duarte Torres, Andreia Oliveira, Milton Severo, Violeta Alarcão, Sofia Guiomar, Jorge Mota, Pedro Teixeira, Sara Rodrigues, Liliane Lobato, Vânia Magalhães, Daniela Correia, Andreia Pizarro, Adilson Marques, Sofia Vilela, Luísa Oliveira, Paulo Nicola, Simão Soares, Elisabete Ramos (2017) Inquérito Alimentar Nacional e de Atividade Física IAN-AF2015–2016, Relatório Parte II (versão 1.1. abril 2017), Porto: Universidade do Porto.
Ludvigsen, Anna and Sara Scott (2009) Real kids don't eat quiche, *Food, Culture & Society*, 12(4), pp. 417–436.
Ministry of Education and Science (2013) *Programa de Generalização do fornecimento das Refeições Escolares aos alunos do 1° Ciclo do Ensino Básico (2005/06 a 2011/12)*, Lisboa: Ministério da Educação e Ciencia.
Ministry of Health (2006) Programa Nacional de Saúde Escolar. *Diário da República*, Despacho no 12.045/2006 (2a série), no 110, de 7 de Junho de 2006.
Morgan, Kevin and Roberta Sonnino (2008) *The School Food Revolution – Public Food and the Challenge of Sustainable Development*, London: Earthscan.
Morgan, Kevin (2014) The politics of the public plate: school food and sustainability, *International Journal of Sociology of Agriculture and Food*, 21(3), pp. 253–260.
Morrison, M. (1996) Sharing food at home and school: perspectives on commensality. *Sociological Review*, 44(4), pp. 648–674. doi:10.1111/j.1467-954X.1996.tb00441.x
Pike, Jo (2008). Foucault, space and primary school dining rooms. *Children's Geographies*, 6(June 2015), 413–422. doi:10.1080/14733280802338114
Pike, Jo and Peter Kelly (2014) *The Moral Geographies of Children, Young People and Food – Beyond Jamie's School Dinners*, Basingstoke: Palgrave.
Ponte, Stefano, Peter Gibbon (2005) Quality standards, conventions and the governance of global value chains, *Economy and Society*, 35(1), pp. 1–31.

PORDATA (2017) Base de Dados dos Municípios, Link: www.pordata.pt/Municipios, accessed on the 3rd August 2017.

Raikes, Philip, Friis Jensen, Stefano Ponte (2000) Global commodity chain analysis and the French filière approach: comparison and critique, *Economy and Society*, 29 (3), pp. 390–417.

Thévenot, Laurent (2001a), Organized Complexity, conventions of coordination and the composition of economic arrangements, *European Journal of Social Theory*, 4(4), pp. 405–425.

Thévenot, Laurent (2001b) Pragmatic regimes governing the engagement with the world in T. R. Schatzki, K. Knorr-Cetina e E. von Savigny (eds.), *The Practice Turn in Contemporary Theory*, London: Routledge, pp. 56–73.

Thévenot, Laurent (2007), The plurality of cognitive formats and engagements: moving between the familiar and the public, *European Journal of Social Theory*, 10, pp. 409–423.

Truninger, Monica, José Teixeira, Ana Horta, Alexandre, S., Silva, V. A. (2013), Schools' health education in Portugal: a case study on children's relations with school meals, *Educação, Sociedade e Cultura*, 38, pp. 117–133.

Truninger, Monica and José Teixeira (2015) Children's Engagements with Food: An Embodied Politics of Care through School Meals, in Abbots, E.J., Lavis, A. and Attala, L. (eds.) *Careful Eating: Bodies, Food and Care*, Farnham: Ashgate Publishing, pp. 195–212.

Truninger, Monica, Horta, Ana, Teixeira, José (eds.) (2014) Editorial introduction: children's food practices and school meals. [special issue on children food practices and school meals]. *International Journal of Sociology of Agriculture and Food*, 21 (3), pp. 247–252.

Truninger, Monica, Horta, Ana, Teixeira, José (2015) School meals in Portugal: governing children's food practices, *Revista de Humanidades*, 25, pp. 31–55. ISSN 1130-5029.

World Health Organization Europe (2006) WHO European Ministerial Conference on Counteracting Obesity. Diet and physical activity for health. European Charter on counteracting obesity. Istanbul, Turkey.

Chapter 5

"Don't bring me any chickens with sad wings"

Discipline, surveillance, and "communal work" in peri-urban childcare centres in Cochabamba, Bolivia

Cara Donovan, Alder Keleman Saxena, Carol Carpenter and Debbie Humphries

Introduction

This chapter focuses on school feeding programmes within child centres for low-income families in the peri-urban region of Cochabamba. Child centres in this region provide up to two meals and two snacks during school days, making them an important source of food in areas experiencing high rates of poverty and malnutrition. However, while child feeding is an important function of child centres in many parts of the world, the social processes surrounding these activities are understudied in the literature. In this chapter, we explore the perspectives of directors and food preparers who are in charge of meal planning and preparation, in order to better understand the social and institutional contexts within which child feeding takes place.

Drawing on surveillance as a conceptual framework, we argue that the Bolivian child centre food programmes examined in this research employ the disciplinary power of the state (Foucault, 1977) to police and modify both administrators' and parents' behaviour. In this system, administrators are instructed to increase or decrease the weight of children based on the results of medical monitoring of the children's bodies. In state-supported child centres, mothers become the subjects of control and surveillance via "communal work" projects, undertaken jointly by the government, centre staff, and mothers.

In practice these partnerships are a form of surveillance and control over both administrators and mothers. Mothers' involvement in the feeding program is tightly controlled by school staff, who manage their participation by imposing expectations, declaring judgments of success and failure, and displaying an overall mistrust of mothers' feeding practices.

While these practices provide conduits for state surveillance and control, they do not guarantee positive human development outcomes. The state does not fully fund the costs of the school feeding programs, which leads to a reliance on the unpaid work of the mothers who are already experiencing the heavy burdens of financial and time poverty. Meanwhile, while administrators are disciplined for failing to achieve, or overshooting, child growth outcomes, they are provided with few informational or material resources to address results of this monitoring. The result is that a system meant to improve the nutritional status of children of low-income families may contribute to rising trends in obesity; and programs meant to support working women rely on women's labour.

Background:
structural adjustment, surveillance, and women's labour

Structural adjustment in Bolivia

Like many Latin American countries, Bolivia was the target of neoliberal economic reforms in response to economic recession in the 1980s. This recession, caused in part by an over-reliance on foreign debt, was coupled with the highest and most rapid inflation in Latin American history (Sachs, 1987). In general, a key component of economic reforms prescribed by international lending institutions was divestment in the public sector. Known as structural adjustment, these policies included the cutting back of state-owned companies, particularly in the mining sector of Bolivia (Draper and Shultz, 2009) and cuts in programs that benefit the poor. The latter included cuts in subsidized food and health care (Schroeder, 2000). Rural agricultural communities in Bolivia were also hit by these policies, when price controls ended and tariffs were cut on foreign imports. As a result, consumers paid lower prices for food, but Bolivian farmers unable to compete with foreign imports saw their agricultural incomes decline (Draper and Shultz, 2009).

In the wake of these reforms, Bolivia experienced a loss of jobs in the formal sector as mines were closed, and a corresponding explosion in the informal sector. Major cities saw a boom in street vendors selling, "an oversupply of cheap imported manufactured goods, from battery chargers and shoelaces to shoes and television antennae" (Draper and Shultz, 2009). As the informal sector absorbed the primarily male workforce laid off in the closing of certain industries, women were also forced to enter the workforce to make up for the lost income of male household members (Schroeder, 2000).

Structural adjustment policies also had effects at the institutional level, principally in terms of the transfer of formerly state-run programs to the hands of NGOs, churches, and private, non-state entities. While these changes were pitched in terms of a broader framework of "decentralization," they had the effect of devolving state responsibilities over education, healthcare, and other services to local level organizations, in many cases without fully developing local capacities to cover these needs (Gill, 2000). Recent years have seen major changes in Bolivian political and economic organization, exemplified by the program of economic nationalization undertaken by Evo Morales Ayma, the nation's first indigenous president. However, as Hindrey (2013) observes, the Morales' government inherited an institutional structure heavily shaped by the neoliberal period, which continues to influence the development of state policies. Much research has explored the impacts of structural adjustment policies on women in low-income countries, (Due and Gladwin, 1991; Geisler, 1992; Sadasivam, 1997; Tanski, 1994 in Schroeder, 2000) concluding that women "have had to shoulder the heaviest burden of poverty and stress resulting from cutbacks in public expenditure" (Schroeder, 2000). This burden was particularly acute in Bolivia, which historically had a large public sector (Afshar and Dennis, 1991). Ameliorating the impacts of poverty on women has been a central initiative of development agencies in Bolivia, including child centres. In particular, the World Bank has been a major source of funds for childcare programmes in Bolivian cities (Schroeder, 2000).

School feeding is an integral part of these programmes. The goals of school feeding programmes vary, but often include improvement in physical, cognitive and psychosocial health. They range from relieving hunger, decreasing micronutrient deficiencies, improving growth, enhancing cognitive development and academic achievement in both higher and lower income countries (Kristjansson et al., 2007). For example, in schools overseen by the Bolivian social services department, the stated objectives include the four "fundamental pillars" of education, health, nutrition, protection, which are facilitated by working with families and the provision of dry food (Secretaria Departamental de Desarrollo Humano Integral, no date). Thus, these programmes are meant to support women working in poverty and improve the health of their children.

The child centres also offer meetings and workshops for mothers on health-related topics such as child feeding. In NGO-sponsored centres, staff make monthly home visits to check on the development of children and educate mothers on topics of health and safety.

Childcare institutions and surveillance

This chapter draw from literature on the surveillance of children and parents in childcare settings, especially Foucault's concepts of surveillance and disciplinary power. Foucault argues that power is exercised through constant surveillance and monitoring rather than an overt display of force. Behaviour of the subject is constrained by making it more visible through techniques of surveillance. He explains how a network of surveillance is used to generate hierarchical power in Discipline and Punish (1977):

For although surveillance rests on individuals, its functioning is that of a network of relations from top to bottom, but also to a certain extent from bottom to top and laterally; this network "holds" the whole together and traverses it in its entirety with effects of power that derive from one another: supervisors perpetually supervised. The power in the hierarchized surveillance ... functions like a piece of machinery ... it is the apparatus as a whole that produces "power" and distributes individuals in this permanent continuous field. This enables the disciplinary power to be both absolutely indiscreet, since it is everywhere and is always alert, since by its very principle it leaves no one of shade and constantly supervises the very individuals who are entrusted with the task of supervising; and absolutely "discreet" for it functions permanently and largely in silence.

(p. 176)

Hierarchized surveillance has been a useful framework for understanding interactions between staff and parents in school settings. For example, Crozier describes disciplinary power present in the "partnership" between teachers and parents in UK secondary schools (1998). She finds that partnership is not merely parental support for schools, but acts as a form of control upon parents: "Although teachers talked about partnership as working together with parents, it was in fact based on the teachers' concerns and definition of the situation, a commitment to bringing about parents' agreement with their view or indeed ensuring consonance" (ibid). Any parent not fulfilling school obligations was deemed divergent. In the UK, the disciplinary practices used to ensure disciplinary power over working class mothers focused on trying to get mothers more involved or to get them to "take on responsibilities" (p. 134, 1998). She describes an effort to teach working class parents how to be "good parents" and the practice of monitoring parents' attendance at meetings and targeting those who did not attend.

Schools and childcare institutions then become an entry point for correcting the behaviour of mothers in regards to child feeding practices (see Albon, this volume). Pike and Leahy (2012) describe this as the "pedagogicalisation of mothers," exploring how mothers have become the targets of food education through school systems in Australia and the UK. Such efforts become a "moral enterprise," whereby mothers are "rendered accountable for the decisions they take about how, when, where and what to feed their children" (p. 439). Thus, education of mothers is an attempt to instil self-regulating behaviour among the mothers in order to ameliorate public health concerns for children's nutritional status.

The underlying assumption is that the mothers' behaviour stems from ignorance, rather than the many complex structural causes or the child's food preferences. The belief that certain groups need education for behaviour change, "fosters a practice of blaming individuals, and fails to consider sociocultural worlds that contribute to individuals' practices of the self" (Lupton, 1996 in Welch et al., 2012). Surveillance of parents by school administrators, and disciplinary power enacted through "participation" and training, thus become ways of bringing mothers' parenting behaviour into line with the State's desired practices, and instilling new, more manageable subjectivities in mothers.

Women's work

In addition to power dynamics present in child centre feeding programmes in Bolivia, this chapter explores these centres' contribution to the time burden on low-income women. In a study of the allocation of time to paid and unpaid work in Bolivia, researchers found that women, on average, work 10 more hours per week than men, with more time allocated to unpaid domestic labour. The average Bolivian woman commits 26 hours per week to paid market-oriented labour and 35 hours per week to unpaid labour, whereas the average man dedicates 42 hours per week to paid labour and 9 hours per week to unpaid labour. Among the men, one-fifth reportedly did not do any form of domestic labour (Medeiros et al., 2010).

This disproportionate burden of time on women has been covered in detail by Caroline Moser's research in Ecuador (1993). Defined as the "Triple Role" of women, women's work includes reproductive work (childbearing and childrearing work), work in income-generating activities inside and outside the home; and community work (organizing and participating in a variety of meetings) (ibid). Moser makes the case that structural adjustment programs increase the burdens of women's triple role in Ecuador. First, the cutbacks in health and human services implicitly assume that the activities necessary for maintaining these resources will continue to be carried out unpaid by women. The underlying assumption is that their labour is infinitely elastic, regardless of the way resources are reallocated (p. 174, ibid). In addition, women have increasingly been pulled into productive, market-oriented work. Therefore, poverty may not only be understood in terms of lack of money, but time poverty. This division of labour has been shown to have immediate and long-term impacts on well-being and personal development trajectories (Friedan, 2001 in Medeiros et al., 2010).

Another feature associated with this trend is that only income-generating work is recognized as work:

> Because of its exchange value, with reproductive and community managing work seen as "natural" and non-productive, and therefore not valued, has serious consequences for women. It means that the majority, if not all, the work that they do is made invisible and fails to be recognized as work, either by men in the community or by

those planners whose job it is to assess different needs within low-income communities.

(Moser, 1993, p. 175)

Methods

Study sites: child centres in Peri-Urban Cochabamba

The child centres where this research was conducted fell into two categories: *Centros Infantiles* (CI) or "Child Centres" and *Centros de Desarrollo Infantil* (CDI) or "Centres of Child Development" (see Table 5.1). *Centros Infantiles* are essentially state-supported preschools for low-income families. *Centros de Desarrollo Infantil* are church and NGO-sponsored education and health programmes for children of all ages. The programmes run by CDIs are complementary to school and other child centre programs, so some children attend both types of centres. Given the small sample size, the purpose of this chapter is not to compare the CIs with CDIs. Rather, it is to provide a better understanding of how the two different institutions operate.

Centros Infantiles

CIs serve children up to five years old who are of "limited economic resources in situations of poverty" (Secretaria Departamental de Desarrollo

Table 5.1 Child Centres Overview

	Centros Infantiles – CI	*Centros de Desarrollo Infantil – CDI*
Funding Source	Controlled by government department of social services (SEDEGES)	NGO-sponsored
Food provision	SEDEGES provides "dry" goods 3 times per year including milk, rice, flour, sugar, oil, lentils, tuna	CDI purchases all food
Menu	SEDEGES nutritionists provide monthly menu for al CIs.	Each CDI regional network contracts a nutritionist that provides an annual menu
Parents	• Pay 70–100 bolivianos per month (£7 to £11) • Take turns shopping for fresh food using list provided by school staff • Attend monthly meetings	• Stay home once per month for CDI staff visit • Attend monthly meetings

Humano Integral, no date, translated by author). There are over 360 of these child centres in Bolivia, with 107 in the metropolitan zone of Cochabamba. The schools that were visited for this research ranged in size from 25 to 140 children.

The stated goal of the CIs is to promote "comprehensive child development, strengthen the assessment and application of cultural practices of attention, care, protection and development of skills, potentialities and to contribute to comprehensive development within the community – family approach." (ibid). Additionally, the government agency SEDEGES works with health centres "to ensure the prevention, treatment and the rehabilitation of the health of our girls and boys" (ibid). Some of the schools have partnerships with a church or NGO, which provides additional funding and support.

Children attending these centres receive breakfast, lunch, and an afternoon snack during the five days of the week that they may attend. The menu is created by a nutritionist working for SEDEGES, and elaborated by school cooks or a school administrator. SEDEGES provides "*alimentos secos*" (dry food), three times per year consisting of wheat flour, rice, pasta, oil, sugar, milk, lentils, and tuna or dried beans. Each CI is responsible for procuring their own perishables such as produce and meat products paid for by the fees the parents pay the school on a monthly basis – 60 to 100 bolivianos per month (£7 to £11).

Parents are expected to participate in the operation of these centres in several ways. In addition to paying a monthly fee, parents take turns shopping for produce, which is either daily or weekly depending on the school. Two school staff administrators revealed that mothers are also expected to bake the bread for the school on school premises. Finally, parents are required to attend monthly group meetings with staff. These meetings cover logistical matters as well as chats and lectures on health topics such as nutrition and child hygiene.

Centros de Desarrollo Infantil

CDIs are child centres sponsored by an international faith-based NGO in partnership with local churches. These centres house two programs: *Programa de Supervivencia Infantil* (Child Survival Program, or CSP) for children up to age three, and the Student Centre that holds program for children from 3 to 18 or 19 years of age. Children under 3 attend these centres once per week, while older children alternate days from Tuesday through Friday. The CDIs serve a morning snack and lunch on each of these days. The CDIs visited for this project served anywhere from 300 to 600 children.

Mothers participating in the CSP can enrol during pregnancy, receiving parental education and food supplies. Their children participate in weekly activities with the intention of providing stimulation and developing motor skills. Mothers of children under 5 years old participate in monthly educational workshops. They are also expected to be home for monthly home visits by the centre staff that involve child development monitoring and parent education on topics such as nutrition or fire safety. Although CDIs serve children of all ages, CDIs were included in this study because they serve children under five and have programming for mothers of children under five.

Data collection

Institutional review boards at Yale University and the *Universidad Mayor de San Simón* (UMSS) approved all research procedures (Yale Human Subjects Committee Protocol #1107008769). Due to limited research on feeding programmes for preschool-aged children in Cochabamba, Bolivia, our goal was to conduct an inductive qualitative study on the experiences of food preparers in programs serving children under six years old.

Data were collected from June through July 2015 through ethnographic methods including qualitative interviews with directors and food preparers at child centres, observations in child centre kitchens and dining rooms, and monthly meetings for staff and parents. Interviews were held with food preparers and directors in child centres in the peri-urban southern zone of Cochabamba. The researcher also conducted interviews with mothers of children under 5. The mothers were selected from a sample of women surveyed by Keleman Saxena in 2014. Although not the focus of this chapter, maternal experiences are also included to compare with school food preparer perceptions of household practices.

One of two Bolivian field assistants accompanied the researcher for interviews of school staff, which were held on school premises. Additional

Table 5.2 Data Collection

Participating Child Centres	*Number*
Centros Infantiles (Child Centres)	4
Centros de Desarrollo Infantil (Centres of Child Development)	4
Semi-Structured Interviews	**Number**
Mothers of children under 5	25
Child centre food preparers	5
Child centre administrators or directors	6
SEDEGES Staff	2

interviews were conducted separately with two staff of the *Servicio Departamental de Gestión Social* (SEDEGES), the state level health and social services department in Cochabmaba. SEDEGES oversees government-funded schools for low-income populations in Cochabamba. One conversation was not recorded at the request of the interviewee. The rest of the interviews were audio-recorded and transcribed.

The research team targeted state-run public and state-sanctioned private schools serving children under 5 that were located in a peri-urban area within a 4 km radius of *the Organización Territorial de Base* (OTB or territory) of Tamborada. This geographical area has experienced rapid population growth from rural – urban migration, home to recent migrants from the nearby rural agricultural zone of the Valle Alto. State-run child centres were purposively selected through recommendations from SEDEGES. Privately run child development centres (CDI) were identified via a snowball sampling method (Tongco, 2007), in which the director of one CDI provided the names of additional CDI directors who agreed to be interviewed after speaking over the phone with him. The researcher interviewed a CDI director or food preparer directly in charge of planning and executing meals.

Interviews with school staff covered broad questions about the logistics and experiences of school meal planning and preparation, as well as their perception of child food preferences. Analysis for this research was an ongoing process occurring with data collection following an inductive approach characteristic of grounded theory. Field notes were written after each interview. Transcripts of interviews were open coded using ATLAS-Ti software. The first author identified issues and emerging patterns were categorized into themes (Strauss and Corbin, 1990). The data was compared to relevant themes in literature.

Results

The results are described below. They are categorized in three parts: (1) expectations of parents within the feeding programme; (2) staff members' perceptions of mothers' child feeding practices; and (3) medical monitoring of children in childcare centres.

Expectations of parents

Food shopping – Centros Infantiles

Within *Centros Infantiles*, parents are expected to participate in the work that goes into providing school food to their children. One school director described her centre as "*comunitario*," or communal, in which administrators and parents have shared responsibility for the labour necessary to provide school feeding.

INTERVIEWER: It's the mothers who buy [the produce]?
RESPONDENT: The mothers, because it is a work – it's a communal child centre. The responsibilities belong to everyone. Not only to me, to the educators, not only to the parents or to SEDEGES. It is an all-including work, I mean, all have, the responsibility belongs to everyone.

To do their part, parents are expected to take turns shopping for produce with a list given to them by the school staff. The money for these shopping trips comes from the monthly school fees paid by the parents. Some schools reported having a specific shopping schedule for parents. For example, one CI expects the shopping trip to be done at 5am on Saturday mornings.

The parent has to go at five in the morning because if you go, let's say seven or eight in the morning, and it is very late. Because the vegetables that you buy, you buy a little. But if we go at five in the morning, so we buy an abundance of vegetables. All have to, *sí o sí*.

Sí o sí meaning "yes or yes" is an expression used in Bolivia to express that there is no other option. The school dictates the market where parents may shop and the timing of the shopping. If the parents go too late, there is less produce to choose from, buying from "a little."

One school food preparer at a CI expressed frustration that a mother had brought the food at 10:30 in the morning, too late to give her sufficient time to prepare the lunch for approximately 25 children. The school director stated that was a problem that would have to be discussed with the mothers.

Another CI was also particular about the location of the shopping. Although this school director stated in the interview that the parent may choose where to shop, she was critical of a mother who shopped closer to home.

Yes, they can choose. But nor can they make a shopping trip for me that is too high [in price]. For example, this week I have had this problem. The mother did the shopping from the little market over here. Here in the neighbourhood. And it's supposed that the little neighbourhood market is always more expensive. For the transport. So this is not good. The mother has to know one – how to economize. To know to buy things of excellent quality, fresh. So, a mother does this no? In the family. Economizes. Looks for the best but always a little cheap. And those who buy it here for me, now of course it's much more expensive.

The larger, less expensive market in Cochabamba is *La Cancha*, about a 20-minute bus ride from the neighbourhood.

The expectation that the mother is responsible for this work is reflected in the director's comment on the role of the mother in the household. The assumption is that the mother knows how to buy fresh and affordable produce for her family. Moreover, the staff member specifically refers to mothers when discussing this responsibility. While any parent may be responsible for the shopping, during the researchers' visits, only mothers were observed delivering food to the school kitchen.

The expectation of the mother to know how to properly shop for her child and family was also expressed during a monthly group parent meeting at one *Centro Infantil*. The school director complained to the mothers present about the quality of food that some mothers were bringing to the school.

> It's not to bother the mothers. It's not that we want to bother you. [This] *Centro Infantil* develops the children together with the parents. We want to guarantee that the children are eating well ... don't bring me a chicken with sad wings ... tomatoes that have worms ... if we love our children, we worry about this.

The implication of this statement is that those mothers that have bought produce with worms or thin chickens do not care about their child's wellbeing, and are admonished publicly. Thus, the quality of the food the mothers bring to the centre reflects the relationship of the mother and the child. That is to say, if the mothers cared more about their children, they would bring better quality food.

School fees: Centros Infantiles

Another expectation of parents sending their child to a *Centro Infantil* is that they must pay a fee for each child that attends. Depending on the school, this fee ranges from 60 to 100 bolivianos per month (£7 to £11). Some school staff members described the difficulty of getting the parents to pay the full amount.

> So, the mother for whatever she earns in the market, it's not to say, "now you have to pay 100 bolivianos" for example. It can't be! So we try to for whatever family, adapt to the budget. And sometimes some mothers can't even pay this 70 bolivianos [about £8]. So they come and help in the kitchen. To peel the potatoes, wash dishes. There is always something, various cases. Various cases that can't pay. So one comes or cleans the patio, does whatever thing and the child is cared for.

If the parents cannot meet the monthly payments, it is expected that they will make up for this by working in the kitchen. Here a school administrator refers specifically to mothers that will work in the kitchen if the household cannot afford to make the payment.

Monthly meetings: Centros Infantiles and Centros de Desarrollo Infantil

The interviews with school staff in Bolivia revealed comparable systems of disciplinary practices to ensure that mothers both fulfil their responsibilities and meet expectations of good motherhood. One way in which parents were brought into agreement or compliance with parental norms in this region of Bolivia was through parent meetings. This provided the opportunity for school staff to instruct parents, mostly mothers, on the expectations, including proper food shopping practices. Staff track attendance of the mothers or guardians at monthly meetings and employ punitive measures. For example, the family must pay a fine of 70 bolivianos (£8) if they miss a meeting at the CI the child attends.

In practice, researchers observed that one father in each of the four meetings attended. This was acknowledged by school staff. Specifically, one school administrator alluded to this in a discussion of school parties held for Mother's Day and Father's Day: "What happens with the fathers, you know that the fathers are more reluctant to participate. But yes, some of them come too."

Although the meetings and school events are open to any parent, it is generally the mothers that attend. The meetings served to cover school logistics, or took on the form of a lecture. For example, one CDI workshop for mothers featured a presentation on child feeding practices given by one of the mothers with a child in the programme. She had attended medical school in Cuba, and was living in the neighbourhood. The presentation was given as a PowerPoint. The mother lecturing in this example was introduced as a doctor and therefore expert on the subject. Thus, her authority came from formal education.

Staff perception of mothers

Not only does parental education reveal an assumption of ignorance of the parents, but several statements made by various school staff members also reveal the concern that parents, particularly mothers, are not capable of adequately caring for or feeding their children.

One school administrator explained that if it weren't for the *Centro Infantil* where she worked, children would be vulnerable to neglect.

> This *Centro Infantil* is a social support for the neighbourhood because it's a poor neighbourhood of needy people ... And if the child doesn't stay here, he stays alone in the house with a key. And the mother leaves a little bread, something for him to eat. And the child is alone in the house all day.

Other staff expressed concern over feeding practices in the household. This CI school director commented that they are teaching the mothers about proper nutrition in the meetings:

> And also we are making the mothers aware in the meetings. Because fast food is what the mothers give [them] in the house. They never give [them] quinoa soup, wheat, things. They eat pasta every day, nothing else. Their tea and their bread.

This director justifies the nutrition lessons given to parents by making the generalization that mothers are not feeding their children properly in the home, only pasta and bread.

Another director, in this case of a CDI, had similar perceptions as to what was and what was not eaten in the home.

> Well what we are seeing is that many mothers now because of their time at work, I don't know for the economic situation too, sometimes they are not preparing these foods that are nutritious for the children. And sometimes, they prefer to make quick french fries. And sometimes for breakfast they buy a Pilfruit and give them Chizitos[1], this they are giving the kids. And it's a terrible food … So they could see to prepare a milk, a rice with milk, porridge with milk, their bread. So this we see that they are leaving behind a lot and I believe it would be very good to make mothers aware of the importance of nutritious food that they should have. Including for her too, for her own state, of the child and also for the [child's] development including the intelligence, no? … One must make our mothers aware of the importance of these foods … Sometimes, for lack of time, they only buy [food] in the street, and nothing else.

There are several claims made in this statement. First, that mothers no longer cook nutritious food, that she observes mothers giving their children french fries or packaged cheese snacks. Although she refers to the lack of time and economic constraints, she also makes the assumption that mothers are not aware or conscious of the importance of what she considers to be healthy food. Finally, she expresses concern that this ignorance of the importance of nutrition impacts the child's intelligence in development, a responsibility of the mother.

Mothers' reported behaviour

My interviews with mothers presented a different picture. Out of twenty-five mothers we interviewed, mothers shared a range of feeding practices. Some mothers did share that they no longer served quinoa in the home due to the rise in price.

> Now for the moment we haven't bought quinoa all month. I have understood that quinoa has gone up a lot. So, in this way as my mother

recently died, so we have been left with pure expenses. So I haven't been able to buy it.

She also shared that she did not cook at home often. However, the reason given was not ignorance.

In general I almost don't dedicate much time to the kitchen because of work. I am a single mother so the work is that which, it's that which I have to do for my children. I am like a father and mother so if I don't work, they are not going to have [anything] from anywhere.

When the mother discussed giving her children hotdogs and french fries, she was catering to her children's preferences.

They like hotdogs. This is it. There is no way to get them off of this. "We'll stay here Mami! Buy us hotdogs and french fries!" This is the food that I prepare for you. Even though sometimes there aren't any hot dogs, the money isn't enough. "But Mami, buy it! We'll split [the hotdog]!"

Although it is possible that mothers give packaged snacks and fries to their children, the reasons for doing so may be more complex than ignorance. Like the school administrator suggested, this mother was experiencing both a challenging "economic situation" and a lack of time, but she also responded to her children's preferences.

Interestingly, the same director who criticized mothers for leaving nutritious food behind explained how she has substituted quinoa for other ingredients on the school menu to adapt to the rising price of quinoa. When asked about preparing quinoa for the school menu, she responded:

Now [the price] has lowered. It was really expensive. So for that reason we haven't been able to prepare it much. Now for that reason we were changing it for wheat, for other vegetables ... Look, a pound of rice is 4 bolivianos. This is accessible. We can buy it. But a pound [of quinoa] that costs 10 bolivianos, this is a lot. Now you can't.

School food preparers, like mothers, adapt their food choices in response to fluctuating prices.

Medical monitoring

One practice all child centres that were visited had in common was the annual or twice yearly medical inspection. This involved staff from a local clinic visiting the centre to measure the height and weight of children. This information is reported back to the directors or administrators.

The following quote is from a female *Centro Infantil* director:

> Two nurses and two doctors came. At the beginning of the first week they monitor the children, taking weight and height [measurements]. So then they gave me [the results] and I'm seeing what state the mothers are handing the children over to me. Now it's been 3, 4 months and they came back to weigh [the children]. They're overweight! The children that were totally malnourished last year, they are now overweight. Now this worries me, how am I going to lower the weight of my children? ... Now I'm not giving them three soups; I'm giving them two soups.

She worries about the rising levels of obesity among the children who are between 3 and 5 years old. Particularly alarming is the rate at which the same children transition from malnourished, to obese, according to this teacher. She started to give children 3 bowls of soup, perhaps in response to medical reports that the children are malnourished. She also responds to reports of rising numbers of children with obesity by changing the number of servings they are given. She expresses her anxiety for this double burden of malnutrition – the coexistence of undernutrition along with overweight and obesity.

Another director described a similar trend in obesity among the children at his CDI:

> The doctors are reporting that I have many children with obesity. It has doubled in comparison with last year... The doctors, well they haven't told me directly but they have spoken with some brothers from the church, that there is a lot of rice and pasta on our menu, and very little salad. So because of this we have the result of the medical examination. So it would be good to consider this... I don't know if there is a lot of rice or pasta, it's not good, no? This is what worries me most, no? ... The doctor tells me that they are very fat. That which I would like to do – to look for an equilibrium. An equilibrium so that the children eat well and that they don't get hungry, aren't malnourished. This is my anxiety, my worry about the menu.

This comment illustrates the use of the results of medical examinations to dictate to school administrators how to feed children in their programmes. This director does not want to be responsible for making children obese, nor does he want children to go hungry. He is told to add more vegetables to the menu, but is not given any strategies to do so.

This director went on to say, "So I need the support of a professional person, that can tell me how much I can change, the combinations that I can make in the menu, the changes I can make. The menu is all that I have, no? Because they are reporting obese, overweight children." The implication here is that this is the job of an expert, a professional. There were two women hired to prepare the meals at this CDI, but it seems that these women are not characterized as professional. In this case, he is looking for a nutritionist that he perceives to be expert.

Other staff articulated that they did not feel adequately supported. For example, one staff member of a CI lamented that the guide menu devised by a nutritionist from the government agency SEDEGES was "ideal" but, "*la realidad es otra cosa*" (the reality is another thing). She explained that although milk was on the menu every day, they did not receive enough milk from SEDEGES to serve it daily, nor did they have enough funds to make up the difference. Thus, the staff were provided with information on the nutritional status of the children, but not given the appropriate tools or resources to address it.

Discussion

The research reveals the inadequacy of top-down programming to provide solutions to the complex problem of malnutrition, particularly in the context of the double burden of malnutrition. Surveillance and disciplining tactics – whether enacted by the state in *Centros Infantiles* or the NGO in *Centros de Desarrollo Infantil* – are used to critique both the feeding practices of mothers within the home and of the staff responsible for the feeding programmes. Blame is placed on both mothers and staff, but neither the state nor the NGO provides adequate information or resources to address the problem. The child centres are then left to rely on the time and resources of parents, namely low-income mothers, for the feeding programmes.

Surveillance in child feeding programmes

This research provides an example of the ways in which the moralization and surveillance of child feeding practices described in the introduction play out in the context of Bolivian child centres. The narratives of directors and food preparers illustrate a chain of surveillance and judgment within the child feeding programmes. Within *Centros Infantiles*, the state agency provides a menu guide to staff as well as medical surveillance through height and weight measurements of children. These results are reported to administrators, who are in turn expected to change the menu or feeding practices according to the results. The school staff exercises a form of surveillance on the mothers, ensuring that mothers fulfil their obligations. The behaviour of mothers is managed through public scolding during monthly parent meetings, and fines for lack of attendance. Mothers are judged for failing to fulfil expectations set by school staff, and for assumed child feeding practices.

This judgment of mothers leads to the justification for educating mothers on nutrition and healthy food, assuming that ignorance is to blame for what they perceive to be poor child feeding practices and in turn, child malnutrition.

The programmes visited for this project use a "one size fits all" approach to parental involvement, a practice critiqued by Crozier (Crozier, 2001; Crozier and Davies, 2007). Programme policy prescribes a framework for parental involvement, particularly for mothers. With *Centros Infantiles*, this involves shopping, monthly meetings, and sometimes the baking of bread. In CDI, mothers are expected to attend monthly meetings on educational themes, regardless of their background or skills. With the exception of one CI allowing mothers to work in the school to make up for unpaid fees, there did not seem to be flexibility in how mothers or parents could be involved.

In these child centres, mothers are not only judged for their participation in this school partnership, but also for what the staff believe the mothers are feeding their children. Much has been written on the burden of blame placed on women for "jeopardizing the health, education and potential productivity of future citizens" (p. 436, Gillies, 2007; Walkerdine & Lucey, 1989 in Pike & Leahy, 2012). A CDI director mentioned the importance of food in the development of the child's intelligence, explaining that mothers needed to be made aware of this connection, so that they do not only provide the "terrible" Chizitos or food bought from the street.

This representation of street food or packaged food runs parallel to that of fast food, which Welch et al. (2012) claim is characterized as bad not only for assumed poor nutritional quality, but also because it is prepared outside the home, thus "demonstrating a lack of a caring relationship between parents (particularly mothers) and children" (p. 716, Pike and Leahy, 2012). Therefore, good parenting would be feeding your child porridge or quinoa.

Nutrition has grappled with a problem of the "close relationship between what is 'good' to eat, as in what is nutritious, and, at the same time, what is morally responsible to eat" (p.154, Coveney, 2006; see also Webster, this volume). In the discussion of obesity opening territories for concern, "parents are positioned as protective or neglectful; children are framed as sick, slothful, dangerous, or innocent, helpless victims." While Coveney's analysis centred on the panic of obesity, Bolivian children could be both under and over-nourished by their mothers. The comments made by school staff reveal concerns that mothers are not providing nutritious food, but "terrible food." School staff members position themselves as the protectors of children, by providing nutritious food in the centres, and educating mothers on nutrition (see Truninger and Sousa, this volume).

The assertion that mothers "never" serve these foods, or that they are making french fries and cheese snacks is similar to Murcott's description of the "moral panic" of the decline in family meals (Murcott, 2012). Murcott reports the repeated assumptions of practitioners and activists, but finds equivocal support for these claims of decline in the family meal.[2] More evidence would be needed to support or refute the claims that Bolivian mothers never prepare certain foods in the home. However, the responses to interviews with mothers indicated that some were serving foods such as quinoa in the home. Nevertheless, the school staff members' perception of inadequate child feeding practices by mothers underpins the moral imperative to educate them on proper diets through workshops.

This form of education is similar to the "human development model" described in Lazar's (2004) research on microcredit NGOs in Bolivia. This term refers to capacity training sessions on family planning, nutrition, infant health, women's sexual health, women's rights, self-esteem, and other issues, encouraging women to construct themselves as particular kinds of citizens (ibid). Like capacity building by microcredit NGOs, child centre lectures are delivered as chats to large groups of women, with a "transmissive notion of education," assuming women do not receive the information anywhere else, beginning from a place of ignorance (Lazar, 2004).

Without considering other factors that contribute to the food that is eaten in the household, the effectiveness of education efforts for mothers to change feeding behaviours will be limited at best. It also assumes all mothers have the same habits and must be subject to the same education efforts. Moreover, an emphasis on educating mothers ignores the role of the child centre feeding programme. Rather than addressing the quality of the food or staff training, presumably due to lack of resources, the mothers become the targets for expert "guidance" (see Chapter 1, Harman, Faircloth & Cappellini).

Women's work

The interviews expose a reliance on mothers' money and time to run the school food programmes in *Centros Infantiles*. Rather than partnership, this relationship is better expressed as a form of control over mothers. The mothers are managed and organized by the school staff.

None of the mothers' activities within the CIs were paid. Rather than work, it was characterized as a responsibility associated with the development of the child, which a CI staff called "communal work." Koch describes community-level work done by women in the "public sphere" in Bolivia to be perceived as stemming from their domestic responsibilities for household consumption in the "private sphere" (p. 59, Koch, 2006). Thus, the role of women in these feeding programmes may be seen as an extension of their domestic responsibilities.

It is important not to overstate the case against child centres or feeding programmes. The centres are not simply bad due to the time and resources they take from poor, peri-urban-dwelling Bolivian mothers. These schools take over the role of childcare for working mothers, presumably freeing up time in their day to devote to income-generating work. Moreover, the directors and staff interviewed for this project were hungry for knowledge to improve the school menu and the health of the children. School cooks were eager to ask for advice from the field assistants who were nutritionists, and interviews would sometimes shift into informal conversations about recipes. The staff of child care centres and of SEDEGES cared deeply about the families they served, and we believe were operating in good faith with limited resources. The problem seems to be, rather, that school staff believe they do the job of childcare better than mothers, and that the mothers cannot be trusted to feed or care for their own children appropriately. This is despite the fact that the child centres appear to be failing to address malnutrition, as monitoring indicates a trend towards obesity among children that enter the programs. In addition, the mandated communal work is implemented in a top-down way which excludes the mothers from sharing their knowledge and experience, while relying on their work and time in this child centre–parent partnership. The reliance on mothers' time and resources for school feeding programmes is particularly ironic given the initial goal of funding child centres to help ameliorate the impact of structural adjustment on women.

Acknowledgments

This project builds on food security research in the region conducted by Yale Doctoral Candidate Alder Keleman. Keleman's dissertation fieldwork in 2012–2014 explored the role of agrobiodiversity in household food security in 8 locations. The data for this project results from qualitative research complementing this project.

We gratefully acknowledge the support of supervisor Dr. Daniel Illanes and research associates Fridda Ramos and Marioni Enriquez. We also appreciate the support of host institutions Fundación PROINPA, the Biomedical Research Institute (IIBISMED) at the Universidad Mayor de San Simón Medical School, and the Centro de Salud Universitario Nueva Gante. The views are the authors' own.

This research was made possible by funding from the Yale Sustainable Food Project Global Food Fellows Fund & Overlook International Fund.

Notes

1 Pilfruit is a processed yogurt snack, Chizitos is a popular packaged cheese snack similar to Cheetos.
2 While a "cooked dinner" in Britain refers implicitly to meat, potatoes, and a vegetable (Murcott, 1982), school staff members lament a loss of the traditional foods cooked within the home – quinoa or wheat, for example.

References

Afshar, H. & Dennis, C. 1991. Women, recession and adjustment in the Third World. In: H. Afshar, C. Dennis, ed., *Women and Adjustment Policies in the Third World*, 1st ed. New York: St. Martin's Press, 3–12.

Agadjanian, V. 2002. Competition and Cooperation Among Working Women in the Context of Structural Adjustment: The Case of Street Vendors in la Paz-El Alto, Bolivia. *Journal of Developing Societies*, 18, 259–285.

Coveney, J. 2006. *Food, Morals and Meaning: The Pleasure and Anxiety of Eating*, 2nd ed. New York: Routledge.

Crozier, G. 1998. Parents and Schools: Partnership or Surveillance? *Journal of Education Policy*, 13, 125–136.

Crozier, G. 2001. Excluded Parents: The Deracialisation of Parental Involvement. *Race, Ethnicity and Education*, 4, 329–341.

Crozier, G. & Davies, J. 2007. Hard to Reach Parents or Hard to Reach Schools? A Discussion of Home-School Relations, with Particular Reference to Bangladeshi and Pakistani Parents. *British Educational Research Journal*, 33, 295–313.

Draper, M. C. & Shultz, J. 2009. *Dignity and Defiance: Stories from Bolivia's Challenge to Globalization*. Berkeley, CA: University of California Press.

Due, J. M. & Gladwin, C. H. 1991. Impacts of Structural Adjustment Programs on African Women Farmers and Female-Headed Households. *American Journal of Agricultural Economics*, 73, 1431–1439.

Foucault, M. 1977. *Discipline and Punish*. New York: Vintage Books.

Friedan, B. 2001. *The Feminine Mystique*. New York: W. W. Norton.

Geisler, G. 1992. Who is Losing out? Structural Adjustment, Gender, and the Agricultural Sector in Zambia. *The Journal of Modern African Studies*, 30, 113–139.

Gill, Lesley. 2000. *Teetering on a Rim: Global Restructuring, Daily Life, and the Armed Retreat of the Bolivian State*. New York: Columbia University Press.

Gillies, V. (2007). *Marginalised Mothers: Exploring Working-Class Experiences of Parenting*. Oxon: Routledge.

Hindery, D. 2013. *From Enron to Evo: Pipeline Politics, Global Environmentalism, and Indigenous Rights in Bolivia*. Tucson, AZ: The University of Arizona Press.

Kristjansson, E. A., Robinson, V., Petticrew, M. & MacDonald, B. 2007. School Feeding for Improving the Physical and Psychosocial Health of Disadvantaged Elementary School Children. *Cochrane Database of Systematic Reviews*.

Koch, J. 2006. Collectivism or Isolation? Gender Relations in Urban La Paz, Bolivia. Bulletin of Latin American Research. *Bulletin of Latin American Research*, 25, 43–62.

Lazar, S. 2004. Education for Credit: Development as Citizenship Project in Bolivia. *Critique of Anthropology*, 24, 301–319.

Lupton, D. 1996. *Food, the Body and the Self*. London: SAGE.

Medeiros, M., Osório, R. & Costa, J. 2010. Gender Inequalities in Allocating Time to Paid and Unpaid Work: Evidence from Bolivia. *The Levy Economics Institute of Bard College working paper no. 495*. Annandale-on-Hudson: The Levy Economics Institute.

Moser, C. 1993. Adjustment from below: low-income women, time and the triple role in Guayaquil, Ecuador. In S. A Radcliffe and S. Westwood (Eds) *Viva: Women and Popular Protest in Latin America*. New York: Routledge, 173–196.

Murcott, A. 1982. On the Social Significance of the "Cooked Dinner" in South Wales. *Social Science Information*, 21, 677–696.

Murcott, A. 2012. Lamenting the "Decline of the Family Meal" as a Moral Panic? Methodological Reflections. *Recherches Sociologiques et Anthropologiques*, 43, 97–118.

Pike, J. & Leahy, D. 2012. School Food and the Pedagogies of Parenting. *Australian Journal of Adult Learning*, 52, 434–459.

Sachs, J. 1987. The Bolivian Hyperinflation and Stabilization. *The American Economic Review*, 77, 279–283.

Sadasivam, B. 1997. The Impact of Structural Adjustment on Women: A Governance and Human Rights Agenda. *Human Rights Quarterly*, 19, 630–665.

Schroeder, K. 2000. Spatial Constraints on Women's Work in Tarija, Bolivia. *Geographical review*, 90, 191–205.

Secretaria Departamental de Desarrollo Humano Integral. No date. *Unidad de Atención Infantil Integral a Niñas y Niños UAIN*, pamphlet, Cochabamba, Bolivia.

Strauss, A. & Corbin, J. J. 1990. *Basics of Qualitative Research: Grounded Theory Procedures and Techniques*, Newbury Park, CA: Sage.

Tanski, J. M. 1994. The Impact of Crisis, Stabilization and Structural Adjustment on Women in Lima, Peru. *World Development*, 22, 1627–1642.

Tongco, M. D. C. 2007. Purposive Sampling as a Tool for Informant Selection. *Ethnobotany Research and Applications*, 5, 147–158.

Walkerdine, V. & Lucey, H. 1989. *Democracy in the Kitchen*. London: Virago.

Welch, R., McMahon, S. and Wright, J. 2012. The Medicalisation of Food Pedagogies in Primary Schools and Popular Culture: A Case for Awakening Subjugated Knowledges. *Discourse: Studies in the Cultural Politics of Education*, 33(5), 713–728.

Part II
The home (and beyond)

Chapter 6

Holiday hunger
Feeding children during the school holidays

Pamela Graham, Paul Stretesky, Michael Long, Emily Mann and Margaret Anne Defeyter

Introduction

Research on childhood deprivation highlights the unfavourable impacts of household poverty on physical health, school achievement, cognitive ability, emotions and behaviours (Brooks-Gunn and Duncan 1997; Brooks-Gunn, Duncan and Aber 1997; Duncan, Yeung, Brooks-Gunn and Smith 1998). Importantly, within the childhood deprivation research, food is often mentioned as a critical link between poverty and wellbeing (Golley et al. 2010; Jaime and Lock 2009). In the United Kingdom (UK) policy makers have recognized that various social policies are needed to help children who are unable to access sufficient amounts of nutritious food (Caplan 2016). For instance, across the UK local education authorities (LEAs) deliver free school breakfast and lunch to children who reside in low-income households. Although efforts to feed children are pervasive, a significant number of children still face food shortages when schools are closed for breaks and holidays (Evans and Harper 2009, p. 91; for updates see Long et al. 2016). This problem is increasingly referred to as "holiday hunger" in the academic and popular press (Butler 2014; Children's Society 2014; Graham et al. 2016). And, despite emerging concerns over holiday hunger there is still a dearth of knowledge about the issue.

This chapter begins with an overview of the social, educational and health related problems associated with food insecurity in children, highlighting a need for year-round preventative measures to reduce food insecurity amongst families. The development of UK holiday clubs is then discussed, reflecting on research to date that has examined the impacts of holiday club participation for children and families. The chapter concludes with directions for future research, emphasising the importance of accurate definition and measurement of holiday hunger.

Social, educational, and health related problems faced by food insecure children

As previously noted, deprivation can determine the amount and quality of food children consume, which in turn structures life chances (Duncan,

Yeung, Brooks-Gunn, and Smith 1998; see Donovan, this volume). Importantly, children from low-income households are especially susceptible to the impacts of holiday hunger as the lack of nutritious food can impede their physical and mental development. Currently, one in five UK children live in poverty making the scope of holiday hunger very large (McCall 2016). As previously noted, low-income children are able to receive free school lunches to help reduce their hunger and/or provide them with a nutritious meal. However, the thirteen-weeks of school holidays can be a challenging time for those children who rely on free school meals as a reliable source of food during the school year (O'Connor, Wolhuter and Every 2015, p. 5). Children that face hunger and poor nutrition during the school holidays may develop a myriad of social, educational and health problems. These problems can impact children's lives and future development and adds to the well-established research on the reproduction of social class and health (Palloni, Milesi, White and Turner 2009). While many problems associated with the lack of food fall within one of these three categories, they impact children in multiple ways (see Truninger and Sousa, this volume). We now review some previous work that highlights the social, educational and health related problems faced by children who suffer from holiday hunger.

Children who do not receive enough to eat often face a decline in general social skills including having problems with everyday interactions. For example, research has demonstrated that hungry children have increased levels of off-task, irritable, aggressive and oppositional behaviours (Golley et al. 2010; Kleinman et al. 1998). Similarly, research suggests that there is an association between hunger and increases in internalizing (e.g. social withdrawal, anxiety) and externalizing (e.g. aggression) behaviours in children (Slopen et al. 2010; et al., 2002) . The social problems that hungry children face are not limited to the direct impacts of hunger on behaviour. Gill and Sharma (2004) suggest that in situations where parents struggle to find enough food for their own children to eat, this can also impact their child's socialising opportunities outside of school. Children may be hesitant and/or refuse to invite other children over to their houses to play when the family does not have enough food to offer to the visiting children. Children may also be worried that once others are exposed to their household economic and food situations, people may view them as poor (Connell et al. 2005).

The social problems that hungry children face can also impact their performance in school. Children who are hungry more frequently fall behind academically, particularly in maths and spelling (Jyoti et al. 2005). They also find it more difficult than non-hungry children to maintain self-control, form and maintain friendships and show sensitivity to others (Jyoti et al. 2005), which are as much social problems as they are educational problems. Research has also shown that during the school holidays, the decreases in structured activity that children engage in compared with term-time can negatively affect children's learning and attainment (Martinez-Lora and

Quintana 2015). Clearly, children who come from food insecure households are at a disadvantage academically to students whose families are food secure. Recent research in the UK has started to focus on the ways in which school holidays, particularly the extended summer break, might exacerbate these issues. In a recent study by Shinwell and Defeyter (2017) the phenomenon of "summer learning loss" was investigated. Data collected from children aged 5–10 years residing in low income areas of the North East of England and Scotland showed that their spelling performance declined significantly following the summer break. This is the first study in the UK to evidence summer learning loss, but the findings support previous studies from the USA and Europe, which have also shown that the school holidays can be detrimental to children's attainment (Cooper et al. 1996; Verachert et al. 2009).

Hunger also affects children's physical health (Cook et al. 2004; Kirkpatrick, McIntyre and Potestio 2010). Hungry children are more susceptible to weight gain because they eat primarily unhealthy cheap food, rather than more expensive fruits, vegetables and lean protein (FRAC 2012; Moreno et al. 2013; Swinburn et al. 2004). Furthermore, research has demonstrated that food insecure children have a higher prevalence of dental caries (Chi et al. 2014), have frequent headaches and stomach aches (Alaimo, Olson and Frongillo 2001), have higher prevalence of chronic illnesses (Weinreb et al. 2002) and often have poorer health outcomes during adulthood (Vereecken et al. 2004). Along those lines, Cook et al. (2004) found that children from food insecure households are more likely to be hospitalized compared with children who are not food insecure. Research also suggests that children who suffer from food insecurity are more sedentary and often do not engage in enough physical activity (Harrold 2016), which encourages weight loss and blood pressure reduction (Janssen and LeBlanc 2010). Children who have food available to them at school increase their intake of healthy food (Murphy et al. 2011) and vitamins and minerals (Gleason and Suitor 2002). Conversely, children who grow up in food insecure households may carry the unhealthy eating habits that they were subjected to as children into adulthood (Hill et al. 2016).

Food insecurity also has detrimental effects on children's mental health. For example, food insecure children suffer from increases in anxiety, depression and other forms of psychiatric distress (Weinreb et al. 2002). Weinreb et al. (2002, p. 7) suggest possible explanations for why hunger affects the mental health of children.

> Food deprivation may result in physiologic or emotional changes that compromise children's mental health or ability to cope with stress. Children may also experience anxiety as a result of unpredictable and intermittent meals. Not knowing whether food needs will be met day to day can result in substantial stress.

Clearly, stress that results from hunger can have a damaging impact on children. Mental health problems often affect other aspects of children's lives. For example, these mental health issues are intertwined with the behavioural problems discussed earlier such as aggression, irritability and an inability to make and maintain friendships. Mental health issues faced by hungry children can be quite serious. Alaimo et al. (2001) found that food insecure adolescents were more likely to meet the diagnostic criteria for dysthymia and more likely to have made a suicide attempt compared to non-food insecure adolescents. In sum, hungry children have to deal with many inter-related social, educational and health concerns that impact them while they are still in school and into the future. We now turn to a discussion of programmes that have been developed in the UK to battle childhood hunger during the school holidays.

The rise of holiday clubs

Food insecurity is increasing across the UK (Centre for Economics and Business Research 2013). This has led many food insecure households to turn to foodbanks to help feed their families (Caplan 2016). The Trussell Trust, a charitable organisation that runs over 400 foodbanks in the UK, has distributed 519,342 three-day emergency food parcels to people in crisis during the six-month period between April and September 2016. Furthermore, 188,500 of those parcels have been given to children (Trussell Trust 2016a). This level of need forecasts to the largest number of food parcels distributed in the 12-year history of the Trussell Trust (Trussell Trust 2016a). Foodbank use rises during the school holidays as, "more than a quarter of parents suffering from some form of food poverty said they were unable to provide food for all the meals their children need during the school holidays" (Trussell Trust 2016b), leading many parents to turn to foodbanks to feed their families. This rise in foodbank use illustrates the need to address holiday hunger in UK communities.

In recent years, a number of other schemes have been implemented across the UK to tackle the issue of holiday hunger by focusing on children more directly. While there have been calls for the UK Government to take action to address the hardship faced by many families during the school holidays (All Party Parliamentary Group on Hunger 2016; Holiday Hunger Task Group 2015; Machin 2016), holiday schemes are currently provided at a local level by various industry, community, charity and educational organisations. There is therefore some variability between schemes in terms of the way they are delivered and where they take place but in general there tends to be a focus on the provision of food and activities in order to reduce inequalities for children and families, particularly those entitled to free school meals (Holiday Hunger Task Group 2015).

Since 2011, the charity Make Lunch has set up over 40 lunch kitchens to provide hot meals to families throughout the school holidays across England, Scotland and Wales. The kitchens are run by volunteers in church, school and community venues and their availability is determined by the individual organisations running the kitchens and what they can feasibly offer throughout the year. The overall aim of Make Lunch is to provide meals to those children considered to be most in need. However, activities such as crafts and games are sometimes offered alongside meals (www.makelunch.org.uk/what-were-doing-about-it).

More recently, as part of their Give a Child a Breakfast campaign, the cereal manufacturer Kellogg's has worked with numerous community organisations to implement one of the country's first holiday breakfast schemes spanning multiple areas across the UK (http://forevermanchester.com/breakfast-clubs/). Through this scheme, children and families are provided with a range of breakfast foods including cereals, fruits and juices, which can be accessed through local community venues such as church halls and community cafés. The breakfast clubs are typically offered universally free of charge to anyone who wishes to attend and often run alongside other enrichment activities such as crafts and sports that breakfast club attendees can get involved in. Like Make Lunch, the provision of a healthy meal is the focus of the scheme while individual clubs determine availability and activities.

Subsequently, schemes have been set up to incorporate the provision of breakfast *and* lunch alongside enrichment activities. Beginning in 2015, Food Cardiff's Summer Holiday Enrichment Programme drew on the support of local schools to implement a four-week project to provide breakfast, lunch and activities for children and families. The holiday clubs were open for 3 days per week, with provision being made available to children for only two days of the week and a family meal organised for the third day where parents could join their children for lunch at school. Various activities such as sports and crafts were also made available to educate children about good health and nutrition and to promote physical activity during the school holidays. In addition, support was given to an established sports programme that had been providing sports activities within the community for a number of years to allow them to extend their provision by offering food to children in attendance. At the same time, as part of a separate scheme, the food distribution company, Brakes, provided support to various holiday clubs across England, Scotland and Wales to allow them to provide nutritious food alongside activities to families free of charge throughout the holidays. Brakes subsequently went on to work with 10 delivery partners, including community and faith-based organisations, to support 142 holiday clubs in 2017 through their Meals and More programme.

With growing poverty rates and greater awareness of the issue of holiday hunger, various organisations have adopted different aspects of the holiday club models in an effort to address the needs of people in their localities. For example, in the summer of 2016, Hartlepool Borough Council invested £25,000 in supporting 18 community schemes to provide food alongside existing summer holiday activities. An additional £13,000 was invested in a scheme to provide food parcels during the school holidays to those families who would usually have access to free school meals during term time. The demand for the scheme was reported to be so high that the planned provision ran out before the scheduled end date, requiring more resources to be made available to ensure the scheme could continue (www.hartlepoolmail.co.uk/news/hartlepool-holiday-hunger-pilot-scheme-continues-after-supplies-ran-out-1-8091819).

Most recently, in January 2017, Mayor's Fund for London rolled out the Kitchen Social programme, which has provided food and activities to children across 23 London Boroughs. The scheme is set to involve more communities over the next three years (www.mayorsfundforlondon.org.uk/kitchen-social-great-things-to-eat-and-do/). Also, in 2017, the charity StreetGames launched their Fit and Fed campaign with the aim of providing food and activities to children in local communities to reduce hunger, inactivity and isolation during the school holidays (www.streetgames.org/fandf/fit-and-fed). Further holiday provision has also been supported through co-ordinated efforts of Sustain and Children North East supported by Big Lottery and in Scotland by Children in Scotland working with Business in the Community Scotland and Brakes.

While the provision of food to support those families considered to be most in need during the school holidays appears to be growing across the UK, it has been argued that more investment is needed to support further development of such schemes. Frank Field MP recently proposed that revenue from the Soft Drinks Industry Levy, popularly known as the "Sugar Tax" (www.gov.uk/government/news/soft-drinks-industry-levy-12-things-you-should-know), should be invested in the extension of free school meals to support families during the school holidays. Working with academics, industry, charity and policy representatives, the All Party Parliamentary Group for Hunger, led by Frank Field, produced a report highlighting the issue of holiday hunger (Forsey 2017). This report led to the development of the School Holiday (Meals and Activities) Bill 2017–19, which calls on Government to take action to tackle holiday hunger on a larger scale (https://services.parliament.uk/bills/2017-19/schoolholidaysmealsandactivities.html). The Government has since committed to the implementation and evaluation of pilot holiday clubs, which will run in 2019. With rates of poverty predicted to increase, it could be argued that holiday food provision would ensure continuity between term time, when free school meals are available, and school holidays for those families most in need of support.

Drawing on evidence from recent evaluations of schemes organised by Kellogg's, Brakes and Food Cardiff, three key themes that have emerged across these studies are subsequently outlined. These themes highlight important considerations for researchers, practitioners and policymakers interested in the development, implementation and impacts of holiday club provision.

Summary of research methods

The research findings subsequently presented in this chapter bring together key themes that have emerged from three studies, which had the overarching aim of investigating the differences that holiday clubs make to children and families. Study 1 was an evaluation of Kellogg's holiday breakfast clubs (Defeyter et al. 2015), which drew on the qualitative views of 17 children, 18 adult attendees and 15 holiday club staff. Data were collected through one-to-one interviews with adults and focus groups with children. Studies 2 (Graham et al. 2016) and 3 (Long et al. 2018) involved holiday clubs organised by Brakes and Food Cardiff. Study 2 data were collected through interviews with 14 holiday club staff. All qualitative data from Studies 1 and 2 were transcribed verbatim and subject to thematic analysis (Braun & Clarke 2006) to consider the differences that holiday clubs make to children and families during the school holidays.

Data for Study 3 were collected from 38 parents whose children attended holiday club. Parents completed a questionnaire booklet, providing information on demographics, their views on holiday clubs and their household food security status. Statistical analyses were conducted to investigate whether households of children attending holiday clubs are likely to experience food insecurity and whether holiday clubs could help to alleviate this.

All studies received full ethical approval from Northumbria University Ethics Committee and informed consent was obtained from all participants prior to study participation. Full methodological details for each study are available in Defeyter et al. (2015); Graham et al. (2016) and Long et al. (2018).

Key themes

Reliable food provision

Food insecurity during the school holidays is an issue that leads to parents adopting a variety of strategies to ensure that their children are satiated, including skipping meals themselves and sacrificing the nutritional value of food in favour of cheaper food options. The provision of food throughout the school holidays alleviated some of the pressures faced by families by ensuring they had access to a reliable and varied source of nutritious food.

> The day before pay day can be tough as you know and it's – [holiday club] don't run out, they don't run out of cereal or they don't run out of milk or they don't run out of bread and so [children have] got the choice there all the time whereas they wouldn't necessarily at home.
>
> (Quote from parent; Study 1)

The alleviation of food insecurity through holiday clubs was further supported by Study 3. Of the 38 parents who responded to the questionnaire, 42% reported experiencing food insecurity during the previous 12 months. Further analysis revealed that these parents were significantly more likely than food secure parents to agree with the statements "Without the holiday club it's harder to make ends meet during the summer" and "Without the holiday club we sometimes find ourselves without enough money for food during the summer". Interestingly, all parents, regardless of food security status, agreed that without the holiday club they would spend more money on food during the summer than during the school year, demonstrating that higher food costs during the summer are felt by all families. However, for food insecure families, this increase in food costs is more likely to lead to meal skipping and hunger than it is for food secure families.

Provision of activities and social support

Whilst the main focus of holiday club provision tends to be on food, the benefits of holiday clubs extend beyond the alleviation of food-related issues alone with the social and support elements of the schemes being highly valued.

The school holidays, particularly the extended summer break, can lead to a lack of engagement in activities outside of the home and subsequent isolation for children and parents. Holiday clubs helped to reduce this susceptibility to sedentary behaviour and isolation by providing families with an accessible place to go where activities are available free of charge. Holiday club participation allowed children to form new friendships and to meet up with peers from school that they would be unable to spend time with otherwise. Similarly for parents, holiday clubs afforded them opportunities to socialise with people from their local community that they would not typically encounter in any other setting.

Although activity participation was not considered in Study 3, it is possible that those families not encountering food insecurity attended holiday clubs predominantly for the social element. Though further investigation is required to establish the motivational drivers behind holiday club attendance, a parent in Study 1 suggested that holiday club activities rather than food are of most importance to some families:

> It's a chance for the children to catch up with their friends because they've got a lot of friends that come as well and it's a chance for me to catch up with other parents urm I think the breakfast part of it is second to that.
>
> (Quote from parent; Study 1)

In addition, where it became evident that families were facing particular difficulties, holiday club staff were able to signpost them onto other agencies that could help them to address a variety of needs beyond the alleviation of hunger alone. Staff acknowledged that it could be challenging to support parents as they can be reluctant to approach unfamiliar organisations for help. Holiday clubs, however, helped to break down such barriers by allowing parents to access support indirectly through activities primarily advertised for children.

Access for all or targeted support?

Data collected across all three studies highlighted a key challenge for holiday club delivery: If holiday clubs are principally set up with the aim of alleviating hunger, who should be able to attend them?

Despite the apparent benefits of participation, many holiday clubs encountered uptake difficulties, with attendance often being lower than anticipated. Whilst targeted support might help to ensure that those families most in need are encouraged to access holiday clubs, parents and staff felt quite strongly that holiday clubs should be inclusive and work to reduce the stigma and shame associated with hunger and poverty.

> I think we still got a way to go to really encourage those people who need to come I think some people are too proud to say I need this and I would really benefit from this.
> (Quote from holiday club staff member; Study 2)

While less than half of parents surveyed in Study 3 experienced food insecurity, 80% believed that holiday clubs should be available to all families regardless of income. Keeping the clubs open to families of all income levels may help reduce the stigma attached to receiving a "hand out," thereby encouraging more food insecure families to take advantage of the holiday hunger clubs.

Overall, these themes suggest that holiday clubs could help to alleviate holiday hunger, particularly for those families who experience food insecurity throughout the year. However, it is important that implementation and promotion of these clubs is carefully managed to ensure that they are not viewed as provision for the poor. This is particularly crucial as the clubs might also serve to reduce social isolation and sedentary behaviour amongst families during the school holidays, regardless of food security status.

Potential issues and directions for future research

The impact of holiday clubs that combat holiday hunger in the UK is promising. Nevertheless, there are several issues that need to be addressed in the development of research and practice in this field, beginning with suitable definition and measurement of holiday hunger.

No agreed definition of holiday hunger exists and the expression has been used in various public and academic contexts to describe different food related problems. References to holiday hunger in the United States, for example, often refer to service drives that provide low-income residents or the homeless with free meals during the holidays. In one instance a US-based charity known as the United Way (Las Vegas) suggests that "holiday hunger" can be reduced by "the Holiday Meal Box program ... that serve as a small way to bless families who otherwise would have to go without food during the Thanksgiving and Christmas holidays" (www.unitedwaynrv.org/holiday-hunger-assistance). In the UK, the expression is also becoming popular and largely used to describe the hardship that low-income households face when schools are closed and children do not have access to free school meals (i.e., "school holiday hunger"; see Children's Society 2014). For instance, the Northeast Childhood Poverty Commission is a stakeholder group that notes, "holiday hunger is a real problem for families who normally receive free school meals" (www.nechildpoverty.org.uk/holidayhunger). Moreover, Butler (2014) suggests that:

> a handful of charities, community groups and local authorities responding to what they see as a growing problem of "holiday hunger" experienced by children from families grappling with cost of living pressures: low wages, insecure work, benefit cuts and delays, and the running-down of community facilities through spending cuts.

As a result of various uses of the term it is not always clear what holiday hunger is, who is impacted (i.e., children, adults, students, and/or households) and what causes the problem (i.e., lack of access to food in schools, poverty, unemployment, and/or government cuts). Researchers are also slow to define holiday hunger and only a handful of studies specifically reference the term. More recently, researchers have begun to define holiday hunger in terms of food insecurity (see Graham et al. 2016; Machin 2016). Nevertheless, despite this lack of clarity, in the UK the expression holiday hunger is gaining popularity in the news and academia as a means to frame (i.e., see Benford and Snow 2000) the problem of children's lack of access to sufficient amounts of food and a healthy diet. Importantly, this use of holiday hunger is well situated within the larger issue of childhood poverty and deteriorating economic conditions that resonate with many people in the UK.

From a scientific point of view, an operational and established universal definition of holiday hunger is needed if it is to be properly addressed by research. In this chapter we propose that any definition of holiday hunger should be rooted in the concept of food insecurity. While there are hundreds of definitions of food security from which we could draw upon, we focus on the notion that food security in relation to physical and economic access. The World Food Summit (United Nations Food and Agriculture Organization 2006, p.1) suggests that food security is met "when all people at all times have access to sufficient, safe, nutritious food to maintain a health and active life."

In contrast to food security, a household is said to be "food insecure" when the members of that household are unable to "access enough food to meet dietary energy requirements" (Pinstrup-Andersen 2009, p. 5). Consequently, both children and adults who are members of food insecure households regularly do not get the proper amount of nutritious food that is necessary for a healthy life. Scholars have examined the impact of food insecurity throughout North America (Blumberg et al. 1999; Coates et al. 2007; Hamilton et al. 1997; Tarasuk 2001; Tarasuk and Beaton 1999), finding that while household food insecurity can be reduced with the help of charitable organisations who provide low-income families with food assistance, it is difficult to overcome the effects of poverty on food insecurity. Food insecurity is also examined in the UK (e.g. Graham et al. 2016), with preliminary results suggesting that clubs that provide children with free food during the school holidays are making positive inroads on reducing food insecurity (Long et al. 2018).

Based on food insecurity research and the framing of children's lack of food during school holidays we propose that *holiday hunger is a condition that occurs when a child's household is, or will, become food insecure during the school holidays*. There are two important aspects to our holiday hunger definition. First, we depart from the US conception of the term that examines hunger in relation to major Christian holidays and focus exclusively on the households of children who are not in school as a result of holidays (e.g., summer holiday). This focus is largely consistent with the use of the term across the UK. Second, we reference households rather than individuals because that is the unit at which food insecurity is measured. Briefly, food insecurity is often measured at the household level to determine if a household can be classified as food insecure (Blumberg et al. 1999). As a result, we suggest modifying standard food security questions as developed by Hamilton et al. (1997) and modified by Blumberg et al. (1999) in the Household Food Insecurity Access Scale (see also Coates, Swindale and Bilinsky 2007). These five questions are amended to focus specifically on the issue of holiday hunger and listed in Table 6.1.

The holiday hunger questions listed in Table 6.1 can be used to create an ordinal scale variable that ranges from 0 to 5. A score of 0 indicates that a household does not suffer from holiday hunger. Holiday hunger increases, however, as the total number of affirmative responses to the questions in Table 6.1 increase. Thus, the higher the score, the greater level of holiday

Table 6.1 Five Questions That Measure Holiday Hunger

1. "The food that we bought just didn't last, and we didn't have money to get more." Was that often, sometimes, or never true during your child's most recent school holiday?
2. "We couldn't afford to eat balanced meals." Was that often, sometimes, or never true during your child's most recent school holiday?
3. During your child's most recent school holiday did you or other adults in your household ever cut the size of your meals or skip meals because there wasn't enough money for food?
4. During your child's most recent school holiday did you ever eat less than you felt you should during school holidays because there wasn't enough money for food?
5. During your child's most recent school holiday, were you ever hungry but didn't eat because there wasn't enough money for food?

Source: modified based on Blumberg et al. (1999).

hunger a household faces. Importantly, these questions tap food insecurity with and without hunger (Blumberg et al. 1999). We focus on households because any measure of holiday hunger must account for the way children are fed in combination with how the adults in struggling households are also significantly impacted. For instance, parents who are able to adequately feed their families through the school year with the aid of free school meals may find it very difficult to continue do so during the summer holidays when free school meals are unavailable. Consequently, parents are forced to buy cheap, unhealthy food to feed their children, and often have to forgo meals themselves to ensure that their children have enough to eat (Gill and Sharma 2004). Some parents are even forced to avoid paying their utility or other bills to have money to purchase food for their children (Drewnowski and Barratt-Fornell 2004). The questions in Table 6.1 modify food security questions by Blumberg et al. (1999) and apply them to school holidays while taking these household impacts into account.

The definition and measurement of holiday hunger are critical at the current time when no specific data on the scale of holiday hunger in the UK exist. However, further to proposing that there is a need for holiday hunger to be defined, it is important that the term is used carefully in practical settings to avoid an association between holiday club access and the stigmatised status of hunger, particularly as the research outlined in this chapter shows that activities are also a central part of holiday club provision.

More research is needed to determine the extent to which these clubs are seen as stigmatizing poverty. This is important because the stigmatization of clubs may lead to segregation and social exclusion (Reutter et al. 2009). If clubs are under financial pressure, it is likely that these community organizations may find themselves limiting access to clubs to more affluent children. Thus, while limiting club access may solve financial pressure for service delivery it may have the unintended consequence of intensifying the stigma of clubs and driving some children who may benefit from the clubs away while simultaneously isolating poor children and shoring up the idea that poverty is largely a personal trouble as opposed to a social problem.

Due to a lack of available data on holiday hunger, it is not clear whether holiday clubs are operating in local authorities where the need for support is greatest. Moreover, data on childhood deprivation is inconsistent across England, Scotland, Ireland and Wales. Despite data limitations, information on childhood deprivation can be compared across England and Wales. The Income Deprivation Affecting Children Index (or ICACI) is an indicator of childhood deprivation collected by the Department for Communities and Local Government (2015). That index is based on the percentage of children in a neighbourhood who are under 16 years of age and living in an income-deprived household (Department for Communities and Local Government 2015, p.27). At the local authority level, the ICACI score measures the proportion of neighbourhoods within a local authority that fall into the top ten percent of the most deprived neighbourhoods nationally. Thus, the index gives some indication of which local authorities face the most childhood deprivation and therefore the most likely highest rates of holiday hunger. The ICACI defines a child's household as income deprived if they receive "Income Support, Job Seekers Allowance, Pensions Credit; or those not in receipt of these benefits but in receipt of Working Tax Credit or Child Tax Credit with an equivalised income below 60 per cent of the national median before housing costs" (Department for Communities and Local Government 2015, p.29). These data can be used to see if there is any overlap between childhood deprivation scores and holiday club programs at the local level. Figure 6.1 shows the 2015 IDACI scores for local authorities plotted against the location of holiday clubs in England and Wales in 2016. Data on clubs was acquired through a national survey (Mann and Defeyter 2016).

As Figure 6.1 suggests, there is an association between childhood deprivation in 2015 and holiday clubs in 2016 across England and Wales. That is, many clubs are located in those authorities where a greater proportion of localities are facing high levels of childhood deprivation. Unfortunately, there are also many areas of the country that could benefit from a holiday club, but do not have one according to the holiday club census. Thus, clubs may not simply be located according to need. Sociological research tells us that community resources and support are often as important as grievances when it comes to the emergence of local organizations (Jenkins 1983; McAdam 1982). Thus, it is possible, if not likely, that as holiday clubs continue to open they will not necessarily do so where there is the greatest need, but instead where there are sufficient resources and political opportunities (McAdam 1982).

As previously noted, holiday clubs are typically formed and run by local charitable, community or educational organisations and have no directive from the UK government that stipulates where the clubs are most needed and/or what services they should offer. Moreover, clubs often leverage

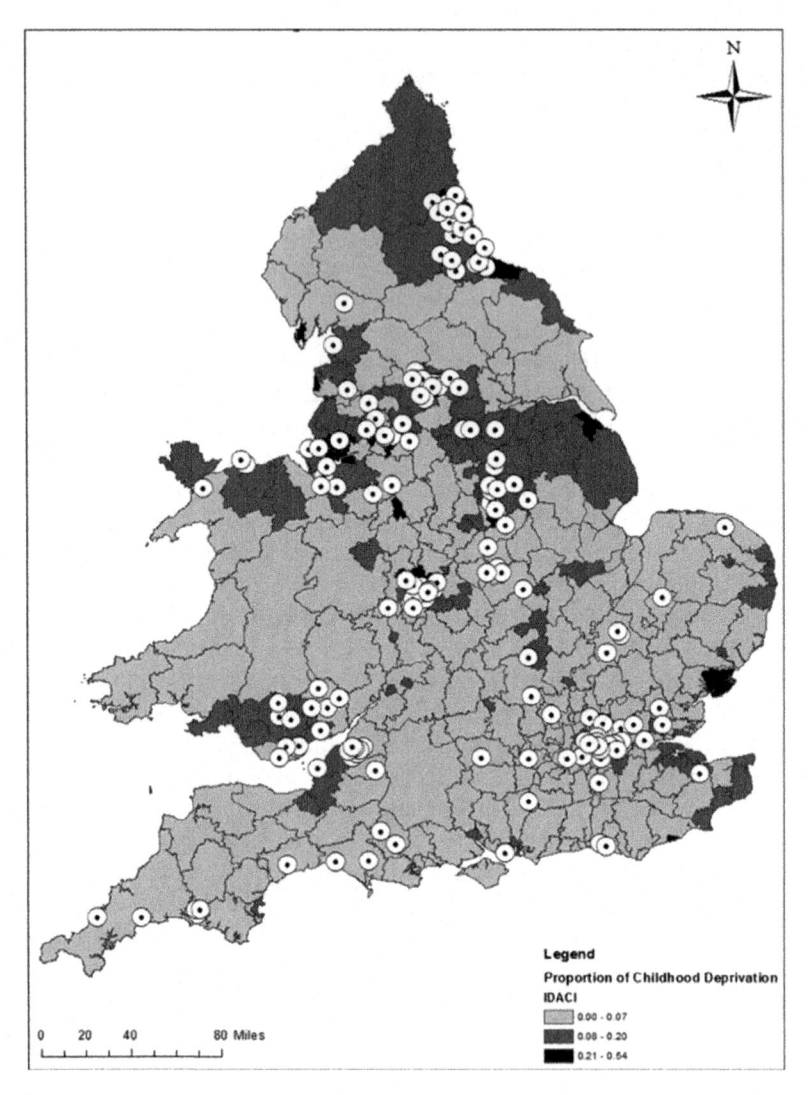

Figure 6.1 Distribution of holiday hunger clubs by childhood depravation in England and Wales in 2016

support from the business sector and the food industry in the form of food donations. Therefore, whether a holiday club exists in an area of need is primarily left up to the community. This formation of welfare services is largely consistent with neoliberal policies that put welfare responses in the hands of individuals (Harvey 2005). That is, the private sector is providing a service at the request of a local community as opposed to that function being carried out by the state. This shifting responsibility from the state to the private sector in order to feed children suffering from holiday hunger may not be the most effective way of distributing resources and may promote a situation that intensifies holiday hunger for the most deprived communities that lack resources to attract third sector investment. A more inclusive, centrally planned approach and funding to ensure equality in the distribution of holiday clubs may need to be examined.

A related issue stems from the widely different offerings in various holiday clubs. Some clubs are open five days a week, while others are only open three days a week. Those that are not open all days of the week may not provide enough relief for families. While clubs that are only open a few days a week do so primarily because of funding and staffing limitations, the children who attend these clubs are receiving less assistance than those at other clubs that are open more often. It is not clear whether clubs in communities with more resources are likely to provide their children with greater access and/or more nutritious food. That is, holiday clubs in the most deprived local authorities may face pressure to cut budgets by reducing the types of food they provide as well as the number of days food can be provided.

Summary

In this chapter we examined holiday hunger in the UK by defining it as a condition that occurs when a child's household is, or will, become food insecure during the school holidays. We suggest operationalizing holiday hunger by modifying five widely used household food insecurity questions developed by Hamilton et al. (1997) and modified by Blumberg et al. (1999). Importantly, these five holiday hunger questions could be employed to obtain better estimates of the level of holiday hunger across UK households with children. Such estimates are not just an academic interest, but also have consequences for the lives of children who live in food insecure households, since there is an increasing need to direct resources that help alleviate the problem.

We also find that children facing holiday hunger are likely to suffer from a myriad of problems (Brooks-Gunn and Duncan 1997). For instance, children who suffer from holiday hunger may fail to develop adequate social skills or act inappropriately in school settings, their educational outcomes may suffer and they are likely to suffer from adverse health. Unfortunately, as childhood poverty continues to increase, the problem of holiday hunger is also likely to intensify. To lessen this problem, holiday clubs have emerged. Initial evidence (e.g., Long et al. 2018) suggests that these holiday clubs may be helping reduce holiday hunger.

As holiday clubs emerge to improve food security in households with children during holidays they face potential challenges that are consistent with attempts to provide services through civil society in the current economic climate. For instance, the implementation of neoliberal state policies has led to an absence of any coordinated welfare effort across the UK. Thus, many communities and local governments are left to solve the problem of holiday hunger by leveraging market forces. For- and non-profit organizations have done an admirable job tackling holiday hunger but these market-based solutions, though well-intentioned, need to be monitored as they may intensify inequality by allowing communities with the greatest need and a lack of access to for- and non-profit markets to continue to suffer. As we suggest, while hundreds of holiday clubs have been established across the UK, more analysis is needed to determine if these clubs are located in areas that have the most need.

Also important is the way these holiday clubs will come to be viewed by those children who attend the club and their communities. As poverty increases there will be pressure on local governments to divert money away from social welfare policies that feed the poor at the same time that demand for these clubs may be increasing. Thus, there is the potential that only low-income children will be allowed to attend these clubs, excluding them even more from the mainstream. If clubs are seen as places for the poor they are likely to be stigmatised and the food security benefits may be offset by social costs.

In the end, holiday hunger is an important and growing public issue facing the UK. Research has not yet adequately defined and examined the problem though existing evidence provides a useful starting point for researchers, practitioners and policymakers. Our intent in writing this chapter is to stimulate more research and interest in the area of holiday hunger, to direct future research and also to help provide information that leads to the establishment of more effective public policy that tackles the problem.

References

Alaimo, K., Olson, C. and Frongillo, E. (2001) 'Food insufficiency and American school-aged children's cognitive, academic, and psychosocial development.' *Pediatrics*, vol. 108, no. 2, pp. 44–53.

All Party Parliamentary Group on Hunger. (2016) *Feeding Britain: A strategy for zero hunger in England, Wales, Scotland and Northern Ireland* [Electronic], Available: https://foodpovertyinquiry.files.wordpress.com/2014/12/food-poverty-feeding-britain-final.pdf, [Accessed: 24 November 2016].

Benford, R.D. and Snow, D.A. (2000) 'Framing processes and social movements: An overview and assessment.' *Annual Review of Sociology*, vol. 26, pp. 611–639.

Blumberg, S., Bialostosky, J.K., Hamilton, W.L. and Briefel, R.R. (1999) 'The effectiveness of a short form of the Household Food Security Scale.' *American Journal of Public Health*, vol. 89, no. 8, pp. 1231–1234.

Braun, V. and Clarke, V. (2006). 'Using thematic analysis in psychology,' *Qualitative Research in Psychology*, vol. 3, no. 2, pp. 77–101.

Brooks-Gunn, J. and Duncan, G.J. (1997) 'The effects of poverty on children.' *The Future of Children*, vol. 7, no. 2, pp. 55–71.

Brooks-Gunn, J., Duncan, G.J. and Aber, L. (1997) *Neighborhood poverty: Context and consequences for children*, vol. 1, New York: Russell Sage Foundation.

Butler, P. (2014) 'Holiday hunger: The charities offering poorer families a lifeline.' *The Guardian* 24 October 2014 [Electronic], Available: www.theguardian.com/society/2014/oct/24/holiday-hunger-charities-children, [Accessed: 15 December 2016].

Caplan, P. (2016) 'Big society or broken society?: Food banks in the UK.' *Anthropology Today*, vol. 32, no. 1, pp. 5–9.

Centre for Economics and Business Research. (2013) *Hard to Swallow: The Facts about Food Poverty* [Electronic], Available http://pressoffice.kelloggs.co.uk/index.php?s=20295anditem=122399, [Accessed: 1 February 2016]. London: Centre for Economics and Business Research.

Chi, D.L., Masterson, E.E., Carle, A.C., Mancl, L.A. and Coldwell, S.E. (2014) 'Socioeconomic status, food security, and dental caries in US children: Mediation analysis of data from the National Health and Nutrition Examination Survey, 2007–2008.' *American Journal of Public Health*, vol. 104, no. 5, pp. 860–864.

Children's Society. (2014) *Feeding Britain: A strategy for zero hunger in England, Wales, Scotland and Northern Ireland*. [Electronic], Available: www.makelunch.org.uk/downloads/Isolation_and_Hunger.pdf, [Accessed: 15 December 2016].

Coates, J., Swindale, A. and Bilinsky, P. (2007) *Household Food Insecurity Access Scale (HFIAS) for Measurement of Household Food Access: Indicator Guide(v. 3)* [Electronic], Available: www.fantaproject.org/sites/default/files/resources/HFIAS_ENG_v3_Aug07.pdf, [Accessed: 17 December 2016]. Washington, D.C.: Food and Nutrition Technical Assistance Project, Academy for Educational Development.

Connell, C., Lofton, K., Yadrick, K. and Rehner, T. (2005) 'Children's experiences of food insecurity can assist in understanding its effect on their well-being.' *The Journal of Nutrition* vol. 135, no. 7, pp. 1683–1690.

Cook, J., Frank, D., Berkowitz, C., Black, M., Casey, P., Cutts, D., Meyers, A., Zaldivar, N., Skalicky, A., Levenson, S., Heeren, T. and Nord, M. (2004) 'Food insecurity is associated with adverse health outcomes among human infants and toddlers.' *Journal of Nutrition* vol. 134, no. 6, pp. 1432–1438.

Cooper, H., Nye, B., Charlton, K., Lindsay, J. and Greathouse, S. (1996) 'The effects of summer vacation on achievement test scores: A narrative and meta-analytic review.' *Review of Educational Research*, vol. 66, no. 3, pp. 227–268.

Defeyter, M.A., Graham, P.L. and Prince, K. (2015) 'A qualitative evaluation of Holiday Breakfast Clubs in the UK: Views of adult attendees, children, and staff.' *Frontiers in Public Health*, vol. 3, p. 199.

Department for Communities and Local Government (2015) 'The English Indices of Deprivation 2015' [Electronic] Available: www.gov.uk/government/uploads/system/uploads/attachment_data/file/465791/English_Indices_of_Deprivation_2015_-_Statistical_Release.pdf, [Accessed: 1 December 2016].

Drewnowski, A., and Barratt-Fornell, A. (2004) 'Do healthier diets cost more?' *Nutrition Today*, vol. 39, no. 4, pp. 161–168.

Duncan, G.J., Yeung, W.J., Brooks-Gunn, J. and Smith, J.R. (1998) 'How much does childhood poverty affect the life chances of children?' *American Sociological Review*, vol. 63, no. 3, pp. 406–423.

Evans, C.E. and Harper, C.E. (2009) 'A history and review of school meal standards in the UK.' *Journal of Human Nutrition and Dietetics*, vol. 22, no. 2, pp. 89–99.

Forsey, A. (2017). *Hungry Holidays*. London: All Party Parliamentary Group on Hunger. Available: https://feedingbritain.files.wordpress.com/2015/02/hungry-holidays.pdf [Accessed: 27 February 2018].

FRAC (Food Research and Action Centre). (2012) 'Hunger Doesn't Take a Vacation: Summer Nutrition Status Report' [Electronic], Available: http://frac.org/pdf/2012_summer_nutrition_report.pdf, [Accessed: 16 December 2016].

Gill, O. and Sharma, N. (2004) 'Food Poverty in School Holidays' [Electronic], Available: www.barnardos.org.uk/foodpovertyreportv3.qxd.pdf, [Accessed: 17 November 2016].

Gleason, P.M., and Suitor, C.W. (2002) 'Eating at lunch: How the national school lunch program affects children's diets.' *American Journal of Agricultural Economics*, vol. 85, no. 4, pp. 1047–1061.

Golley, R., Baines, E., Bassett, P., Wood, L., Pearce, J., and Nelson, M. (2010) 'School lunch and learning behaviour in primary schools: an intervention study.' *European Journal of Clinical Nutrition*, vol. 64, no. 11, pp. 1280–1288.

Graham, P.L., Crilley, E., Stretesky, P.B., Long, M.A., Palmer, K.J., Steinbock, E. and Defeyter, M.A. (2016) 'School holiday food provision in the UK: A qualitative investigation of needs, benefits, and potential for development.' *Frontiers in Public Health* [Electronic] Available: https://doi.org/10.3389/fpubh.2016.00172, [Accessed: 16 December 2016].

Hamilton, W.L., Cook, J.T., Thompson, W.T., Buron, L.T., Frongillo, E.A., Olson, C.M., and Wehler, C.A. (1997) 'Household food security in the United States in 1995: Summary report of the Food Security Measurement Project' [Electronic] Available: www.fns.usda.gov/sites/default/files/SUMRPT.PDF, [Accessed: 16 December 2016]. Alexandria, VA (USA): U.S. Department of Agriculture, Food and Consumer Service.

Harrold, A. (2016) 'PE during holidays needed to tackle children's sedentary lifestyle' [Electronic], Available: www.communitypractitioner.com/news/pe-during-holidays-is-needed-to-tackle-sedentary-lifestyle-of-children-campaigners-say, [Accessed: 16 December 2016].

Harvey, D. (2005) *A Brief History of Neoliberalism*. New York: Oxford University Press.

Hill, S., Prokosch, M., DelPriore, D., Griskevicius, V. and Kramer, A. (2016) 'Low childhood socioeconomic status promotes eating in the absence of energy need.' *Psychology Science*, vol. 3, no. 3, pp. 354–364.

Holiday Hunger Task Group. (2015) *Filling the Holiday Gap Update Report 2015* [Electronic], Available: www.fillingtheholidaygap.org/APPG_Holiday_Hunger_Report_2015.pdf, [Accessed: 24 November 2016].

Jaime, P.C. and Lock, K. (2009) 'Do school based food and nutrition policies improve diet and reduce obesity?' *Preventive Medicine*, vol. 48, no. 1, pp. 45–53.

Janssen, I. and LeBlanc, A.G. (2010) 'Systematic review of the health benefits of physical activity and fitness in school-aged children and youth.' *International Journal of Behavioral Nutrition and Physical Activity*, vol. 7, no. 40, pp. 1–16.

Jenkins, C. (1983) 'Resource mobilization theory and the study of social movements.' *Annual Review of Sociology*, vol. 9, pp. 527–553.

Jyoti, D., Frongillo, E. and Jones, S. (2005) 'Food insecurity affects school children's academic performance, weight gain, and social skills.' *The Journal of Nutrition*, vol. 135, no. 12, pp. 2831–2839.

Kirkpatrick, S., McIntyre, L. and Potestio, M.L. (2010) 'Child hunger and long-term adverse consequences for health.' *Archives of Pediatrics and Adolescent Medicine*, vol. 164, no. 8, 754–762.

Kleinman, R.E., Murphy, J.M., Little, M., Pagano, M., Wehler, C.W., Regal, K., and Jellinek, M.S. (1998) 'Hunger in children in the United States: Potential behavioral and emotional correlates.' *Pediatrics*, vol. 101, no. 1, pp. 1–6.

Long, M.A., Stretesky, P., Graham, P.L., Palmer, K.J., Steinbock, E. and Defeyter, M.A. (2018) 'The impact of holiday clubs on household food insecurity: A pilot study.' *Health and Social Care in the Community*, vol. 26, pp. e261–e269.

Long, R. (2016) 'School Meals and Nutritional Standards' Briefing Paper Number 04195 [Electronic], Available: http://researchbriefings.parliament.uk/ResearchBriefing/Summary/SN041954 [Accessed: 23 November 2016]. London: House of Commons Library.

Machin, R.J. (2016) 'Understanding holiday hunger.' *Journal of Poverty and Social Justice*, vol. 24, no. 3, pp. 311–319.

Mann, E. and Defeyter, M.A. (2016) *Mapping of holiday provision programmes in the UK*. UK All Party Parliamentary Group on School Food Meeting: London.

Martinez-Lora, A.M., and Quintana, S.M. (2015) 'Summer learning loss.' *Encyclopaedia of Cross Cultural School Psychology* [Electronic], Available: http://link.springer.com/referenceworkentry/10.1007%2F978-0-387-71799-9_415, pp. 962–963 [Accessed: 16 December 2016].

McAdam, D. (1982) *Political Process and the Development of Black Insurgency 1930–1970*. Chicago, IL: University of Chicago Press.

McCall, B. (2016) 'Child poverty continues to rise in the UK.' *The Lancet*, vol. 388, no. 10046, p. 747.

Moreno, J.P., Johnston, C.A. and Woehler, D. (2013) 'Changes in weight over the school year and summer vacation: Results of a 5-year longitudinal study.' *Journal of School Health*, vol. 83, no. 7, 473–477.

Murphy, S., Moore, G.F., Trapper, K., Lynch, R., Clarke, R., Raisanen, L., Desousa, C. and Moore, L. (2011) 'Free healthy breakfasts in primary schools: A cluster randomized controlled trial of a policy intervention in Wales, UK.' *Public Health Nutrition*, vol. 14, no. 2, pp. 219–226.

O'Connor, J., Wolhuter, C. and Every, S. (2015). 'Holiday Kitchen. An evaluation of Holiday Kitchen 2014: Learning, food and play for families who need it most in the West Midlands,' *Ashram Moseley* [Electronic] Available: www.familyaction.org.uk/content/uploads/2015/01/hk_bcu_report.pdf, [Accessed: 1 February 2016].

Palloni, A., Milesi, C., White, R.G., and Turner, A. (2009) 'Early childhood health, reproduction of economic inequalities and the persistence of health and mortality differentials.' *Social Science and Medicine*, vol. 68, no. 9, pp. 1574–1582.

Pinstrup-Andersen, P. (2009) 'Food security: Definition and measurement.' *Food Security*, vol. 1, no. 1, pp. 5–7.

Reutter, L.I., Stewart, M.J., Veenstra, G., Love, R., Raphael, D. and Makwarimba, E. (2009) 'Who do they think we are, anyway?: Perceptions of and responses to poverty stigma.' *Qualitative Health Research*, vol. 19, no. 3, pp. 297–311.

Shinwell, J. and Defeyter, M.A. (2017). 'Investigation of summer learning loss in the UK-Implications for holiday club provision.' *Frontiers in Public Health*, vol. 5, no. 270.

Slopen, N., Fitzmaurice, G., Williams, D.R., and Gilman, S.E. (2010) 'Poverty, food insecurity, and the behavior of childhood internalizing and externalizing disorders.'

Journal of the American Academy of Child and Adolescent Psychiatry vol. 49, no. 5, pp. 444–452.

Swinburn, B.A., Caterson, I., Seidell, J.C., and James, W.P. (2004) 'Diet, nutrition and the prevention of excess weight gain and obesity.' *Public Health Nutrition*, vol. 7, no. 1A, pp. 123–146.

Tarasuk, V. (2001) 'A critical examination of community-based responses to household food insecurity in Canada.' *Health Education and Behavior*, vol. 28, no. 4, pp. 487–499.

Tarasuk, V. and Beaton, G. (1999) 'Household food insecurity and hunger among families using food banks.' *Canadian Journal of Public Health*, vol. 90, no. 2, pp. 109–113.

Trussell Trust. (2016a) Latest Stats [Electronic] Available: www.trusselltrust.org/news-and-blog/latest-stats/, [Accessed: 15 December 2016].

Trussell Trust. (2016b) One in Five Parents Struggling to Feed Their Children [Electronic] Available: www.trusselltrust.org/wp-content/uploads/sites/2/2015/06/1-in-5-parents-struggling-to-feed-children-1.pdf, [Accessed: 15 December 2016].

United Nations Food and Agriculture Organization. (2006) Food Security [Electronic] Available: www.fao.org/forestry/13128-0e6f36f27e0091055bec28ebe830f46b3.pdf, [Accessed: 16 December 2016].

Verachtert, P., Van Damme, J., Onghena, P. and Ghesquiere, P. (2009). 'A seasonal perspective on school effectiveness: Evidence from a Flemish longitudinal study in Kindergarten and First Grade.' *School Effectiveness and School Improvement*, vol. 20, no. 2, pp. 215–233.

Vereecken, C., Ojala, K., and Jordan, M.D. (2004) 'Eating habits' in C. Currie, C. Roberts, A. Morgan et al., editors *Young People's Health in Context. Health Behaviours in School-Aged Children (HBSC) Study: International Report from the 2001/2002 Survey. Health Policy for Children and Adolescents.* (Vol. 4), Copenhagen: WHO, pp. 110–119.

Weinreb, L., Wehler, C., Perloff, J., Scott, R., Hosmer, D., Sagor, L. and Gundersen, C. (2002) 'Hunger: Its impact on children's health and mental health.' *Pediatrics*, vol. 110, no. 4, pp. 1–9.

Chapter 7

"My mum feeds me, but really, I eat whatever I want!"

A relational approach to feeding and eating

Zofia Boni

Introduction

Feeding a child, as other chapters in this book show, is a complex act. Feeding requires constant maintenance: planning what a child might eat, shopping for necessary foodstuffs, preparing meals and putting food on a child's plate (or in her mouth), while taking into consideration other members of the family and their preferences, guidelines concerning "proper eating" and various constraints related to time, space and money. Furthermore, these activities are all overlain by numerous influences from various sources that try to regulate mothering (see for example, Cairns et al., this volume). Feeding is a deeply emotional and also bodily, material, cultural, social and political experience. As DeVault explains in her classic book *Feeding the Family* (1991), a great part of the feeding process is invisible because to a large extent it is a mental process. "Producing meals requires thoughtful coordination and interpersonal work as well as the concrete tasks of preparation (...) Feeding implies a relatedness, a sense of connection with others" (DeVault 1991, p. 39). It is that relatedness that I want to focus on here.

During my fieldwork in Warsaw, it became evident that children often do not eat in the exact way in which adults want to feed them. Ideas about, and practices of feeding might and often do differ from those about eating, and *vice versa*; and as they are inextricably linked, these differences cause a lot of tension. One of the mothers I talked to in Warsaw told me, for example: "I can have my ideas about feeding her, but after all, she will eat whatever she wants, the feeding comes down to her eating something." In many families it is more often about non-feeding: avoiding, restricting and controlling eating (of sweets, for example), than actually feeding. Similarly, it is often more about non-eating: refusing to be fed rather than eating. Feeding and eating are entangled in multiple ways. Adults not only feed children, of course, but they also feed themselves and other adults. And children also sometimes feed others or themselves. What is more, the individual actors engaged in feeding and eating are in fact plural, that is they are "not completely 'the same' in different contexts of social life" (Lahire 2011, p. xiii). To give an example, and as this book explores, children eat differently at home and at school. Parents feed their children differently at home and in public spaces. There is therefore a plurality of practices and experiences connected to both feeding and eating.

Since the two are so closely tied, we have to look both at feeding and at eating, and at the relationship between them if we want to understand the complexity of these actions. To understand one, we have to understand the other. We have to look at the actors involved and the processes that shape this relationship. This is what I provide in this chapter, arguing for the relational approach to feeding and eating. The more theoretical considerations discussed below will be followed and illustrated by the ethnographic accounts from my research in Warsaw.

Relational approach to feeding and eating

Inspired by Desmond, I argue for the relational approach in constructing and studying scientific objects (2014, p. 548). Relational approaches to ethnographic research are characterized by studying fields rather than places, studying boundaries rather than bounded groups and studying processes rather than people, and studying cultural conflict rather than group culture (2014, pp. 563–569). When studying feeding, we cannot look only at a person who feeds but should rather look at the whole web of relations and social actors which influence the person who feeds and the process of feeding. This includes children as well.

Feeding and eating are multi-dimensional and entangle many actors in different ways. They relate to both the symbolic and the material dimensions of food and involve both individuals and collective or institutional entities. They engage those directly involved, for example parents and children, but also those involved indirectly, such as food producers, retailers, state authorities and media outlets. In this chapter I limit my analysis to the relationship between parents and children, but elsewhere discuss other social actors and their influences on feeding and eating in Warsaw (Boni 2016).

Feeding and eating could be looked at as one interconnected process, consisting of multiple practices, material objects, symbolic meanings and expectations. Eating, for instance, is not only about putting food in one's mouth, chewing, swallowing and digesting it. Eating is both a conceptual and a physical practice (Abbots and Lavis 2013, p. 4). Strathern points out that "in describing actions, eating also describes relations" (2012, p. 2). Eating is about what is eaten, and how, where, when and with whom is it eaten. On the couch in front of the TV or in the restaurant – these are very different eating experiences. Eating, more importantly, is also about who is feeding a person who eats (as well as how they do it). Strathern explains that "agents know themselves as persons through the food they consume; eating decomposes their multiple relations into the specific axis relevant to the food source" (2012, p. 9). She adds that being fed as a mother is not the same as being fed as a daughter. The way in which children are fed (and eat) identifies them as children and shapes their relations with others (see for example, Boni 2015).

Strathern also points out that eating is an ambiguous experience: "readiness to eat is also a sign that the source of what is to be eaten can be trusted …. Food itself is the result of others' relationships." (2012, pp. 8–9). A child, in particular, is dependent on the feeding practices of others. Eating as a child usually means that you have to trust others and that your daily food encounters are structured by adults who set up many rules related to eating. Being fed by adults usually means being cared for; however, children are not the passive recipients of care. They actively influence the processes of feeding and eating. When I talked to 11-year-old Krzysiek about food and feeding-eating in his family, he told me: "my mum feeds me, but really, I eat whatever I want!" The two are intermingled. Strathern (2012) explains that what one eats is at the same time the outcome of the agency of others. I would add that what one feeds is also the result of the agency of a person who eats, which in the case of children is often forgotten. Agency can be about intentionality of action, about being empowered and "enacting the process of reflecting on the self and the world and of acting simultaneously within and upon what one finds there" (Ortner 2006, p. 57); but is not necessarily always fully "conscious", as many social consequences are in fact unintended effects of certain actions. Agency is also about pursuing projects while acting within the relations of social inequality, asymmetry and force. For children exercising their agency, this often means engaging in resistance practices, but within the scope and the limits that their social position allows (see Marshall, this volume).

Feeding a child is also a gendered experience (see Charles and Kerr 1988; Murcott 1983; 2000). "It takes proper food from the right source to make feeding nourishing" (Strathern 2012, p. 6) and this "nourishing art" – as Giard (1998) calls it – is predominantly a mother's duty. As in many other Global North societies (e.g. Cairns and Johnston 2015), in Poland, feeding is predominantly women's job. The need to feed and nurture is often perceived as an innate biological necessity and is indeed seen as fundamental to being a mother and a woman (see Hryciuk and Korolczuk 2012). While it might feel for mothers that, as Paulina told me, "it is in the maternal instinct: this need to feed", in fact, as DeVault explains, "the activities of feeding the family are of course not really instinctual; they are socially organized and their logic is learned" (1991, p. 48). The caring work, as DeVault continues to explain, is based on putting oneself in another's place and anticipating and understanding their needs, "feeding is finding a balance between the sociability of group life and the concern for individuality" (1991, p. 78). Similar to eating, feeding is an ambiguous experience as it is both about providing necessary and "proper" food – about caring and nurturing – but also about disciplining children and teaching them how to eat (see Webster, this volume).

As I show, parents and children negotiate their feeding and eating, crossing and bending many boundaries and engaging in multiple power struggles (see Grieshaber 1997; O'Connell and Brannen 2014). I find de Certeau's theory and his distinction between *strategies* and *tactics* (1984, pp. 29–44) useful when thinking about these power struggles and family foodways. *Strategies* are implemented by institutions and structures of power – in this case adults; they have the status of the dominant, hegemonic order and attempt to set certain behaviours and courses of action by establishing a panoptic position. Parental strategies to a greater or lesser extent reflect their ideas about "proper" feeding. *Tactics* are much more flexible and are employed by people – in this case children – acting in the environment defined by strategies. They are "the art of the weak" (de Certeau 1984, p. 37). Tactics are developed to evade or negotiate strategies towards their own purposes and desires to create a sphere of autonomous action. This is not, however, a simple binary, strategies and tactics are entangled in many ways and constantly influence each other. Both are embedded in the everyday life and are not necessarily reflexive or overt: they do not necessarily follow the intentional, goal-oriented logic, but can be habitual, following the logic of everyday practice. However, family relations are not only characterized by such a configuration. It is not that parents only strategize, and children only tactfully resist. They also care, love and share, and use food to do that. But strategies and tactics constitute important elements of their family foodways and therefore are vital for understanding the feeding-eating relations.

Research methods

This chapter stems from my doctoral research on children and food carried out in Warsaw in 2012–2013 (Boni 2016). Here I focus on the part of my research which concerned families. I worked with fifteen families, all of whom can be described as middle class, although they varied immensely in terms of their socio-economic situations and social, economic and cultural capitals (Bourdieu 1984). In most of the families both parents were in paid employment and women, with only few exceptions, were also additionally responsible for housework, including foodwork.

I conducted separate interviews with mothers and in few families with fathers. I also talked to several grandparents. I conducted semi-structured interviews, which relate more to people's narratives and what they say they do, than to their practices and what they do. However, as de Certeau explains: "narrativity has a fundamental theoretical relevance to the study of the practices of everyday life" (1980, p. 29). It is one of the ways to learn about people's practices. Moreover, conducting separate interviews with different members of the family, mothers and children, and sometimes also fathers and grandparents, helps to create a more coherent picture of family foodways and family display (James and Curtis 2010). Furthermore, I participated in meals in three households, joining families for different occasions, usually during weekends, be it for breakfast or dinner. Additionally, many of the interviews I conducted – including all of the meetings with children – happened in my interlocutors' homes. I have usually spent at least a couple of hours with each of the families. I was often served something to eat or drink, or witnessed food preparations, which allowed me, if not entirely able to participate and observe, at least to peek into their food lives.

Building on the approach of childhood studies (e.g. Mayall 1994; James, Jenks and Prout 1998), during my research I treated children as independent people, knowledgeable about their own and others' lives. My focus was on children between 6 and 12 years old, which constitutes the age of primary school children in Poland. I conducted semi-structured interviews with them and also used drawing and filling out vignettes as a method of communicating with younger children (Christensen and James 2008). Research with children allowed me not only to find out about their foodways and eating experiences, but also to get their opinions and perspectives on family life and the process of feeding.

Family foodways

I had my first dinner with the Podolscy family on a cold December day. We ate almost immediately after my arrival. The table was set up in their small dining-living room. Małgosia (37-year-old NGO worker) and Mikołaj (38-year-old photographer) were in the kitchen, putting the portions of fried fish on our plates, and then they brought them to the table where I and the children were sitting. I was invited to serve myself, while Małgosia put *surówka* (a salad made from raw vegetables) and boiled potatoes on her children's plates. This was followed by a discussion:

> "No, I don't want *surówka*, I'm not going to eat it", said 7-year-old Bartek.
> "Try at least a little bit. I will give you some. How many potatoes do you want?" responded Małgosia.
> "Fifty spoons, a lot, a lot!"
> "You won't eat so much, I will give you three, and if you want more, I'll add more."

We started eating. One more fish was still in the pan, so Małgosia from time to time went to the kitchen to turn it over. Bartek's younger sister, Zuzia, wanted to change seats, so Małgosia, and later again Mikołaj, switched seats with her. She also complained that she wanted more fish, and more *surówka*, though she still had not eaten what was on her plate. She played with the *surówka* ingredients pretending that they were worms. She put a piece of cabbage under my nose, while asking if I would like to eat a worm. Everyone talked at the same time. Bartek was telling me about his school. At some point he stood up from the table and went to his room to get a book he wanted to show me. His father asked him to get back to the table and sit up straight. After a while Zuzia said that she could not eat anything more:

"Can I go now? I don't want to eat anymore!"
"Eat a little bit more" answered Małgosia.
"But I don't want to."
"You have barely eaten anything."
"I can't eat more."
"Eat a piece of fish and a bit more of *surówka*, and then you can go. You can leave the potatoes," said Małgosia while indicating with a fork on Zuzia's plate what she should eat.
Zuzia put all of it in her mouth at once and left the table.
(All noted in my field notes on 1st December 2012)

This is a fairly typical situation. Parents attempt to feed their children in a particular way while children have their own ideas about eating, which results in diverse verbal and non-verbal negotiations and power struggles. Małgosia wants her children to eat a balanced meal, *a little bit of everything*. But Bartek prefers eating potatoes to eating *surówka*. His attempts to eat a lot of the former, and not eat the latter are restricted by his mother when she puts potatoes and vegetables on his plate. Children not only show their opinions about how much food and what ingredients they prefer to eat, they also demonstrate their other wishes, for example regarding the seat they take. Zuzia changed seats with her parents several times, and they always complied with her demands. However, when her older brother got up from the table before finishing the meal and before being excused to leave, he was instructed to come back.

A parent, usually a mother, feeds a child. She organizes it in the form of a meal. A child eats. Or he does not. This might seem like the simplest, the most natural and instinctive relationship. The basic exchange. The gift of food and care. A mother gives food and organizes the feeding, while a child is expected to reciprocate and eat it. Additionally, it could be argued, it is assumed that a child will take care and feed the mother in her old age. However, when we look at that relationship and exchange more closely, it turns out there is nothing simple about it, at least not according to the people who participate in it.

The feeding–eating relations and family foodways change significantly when children are around. When I asked my interlocutors how their ways of eating have changed when they had children, all of them mentioned that their food habits became much more structured, organised and conservative, in comparison with their chaotic food habits from before having children. They all have a sort of routine family menu, repeated over and over again. Some parents seemed to long for the spontaneous and more laid-back attitude to food, for various pleasures. For example, Małgosia told me that she misses "enjoying a long, calm meal with a glass of wine with [her] husband". They also eat out less, partly because of financial constraints, and partly because going out to the restaurant with children is considered to be rather problematic. However, the situation of eating itself became more chaotic. 28-year-old Kasia, asked about her dream and ideal meal, told me: "that would be a meal eaten not as a mother: calmly, slowly, at the table and not running around it after kids". Mothers often do not have time to eat "properly" themselves. 33-year-old Anna mentioned: "I sometimes feel like a dumpster, I just eat what they have left; otherwise we would throw it away. It's not nice though, to eat such a half-eaten, tossed on the plate meal."

Many parents mentioned that they had more time for cooking before; there was a place for culinary experiments, which according to them cannot take place with children around. For some, however, the change was to have less time for cooking and also the cooking itself becoming rather plain and simple; for others having children was the reason to start cooking at all. 29-year-old Dominika told me:

> Certainly, we eat in a different way! I cook mainly for children, I think of them when I cook. I cook on a daily basis. If I was on my own, I would probably sometimes eat only sandwiches, when I don't have time or when I'm not in the mood for preparing a proper meal, but children motivate me to do that.

Children's eating is seen as more important than parents'. As a result, feeding children often comes at the expense of parental food preferences and habits. Many mothers told me about their favourite food, such as seafood and spicy dishes, which they no longer prepare because their children would not eat them. In that way children's eating (or non-eating) not only influences the process of feeding them, but also their parents' eating.

Family meals in Warsaw are more and more often adjusted to children's tastes and preferences. In the past, the tastes and preferences of men took priority over those of women and children (see Murcott 1983: 2000; Charles and Kerr 1988). But with the emergence of intensive parenting practices (Hays 1996) children often become the main focus of the feeding process, the centre of women's attention.

Organising family foodways and foodwork at home involves additional coordination and strategizing when both parents are engaged in the process of feeding children. In the Podolscy family the foodwork at home is shared. Mikołaj does a large grocery shop during the weekend, and then on

Mondays, Wednesdays and Fridays, Małgosia leaves work early to pick up the children from the kindergarten and school, and she cooks dinner and prepares supper for them. On those days Mikołaj prepares their breakfast. On Tuesdays and Thursdays Mikołaj goes to work very early while Małgosia prepares breakfast for their children, and he leaves work early to pick up the children, take care of them and prepare food for them on these days. Mikołaj and Małgosia implement this elaborate plan in order to coordinate feeding and eating at their home. But they also have to coordinate the process of feeding–eating with their work responsibilities and other factors, such as opening times of educational institutions. Many parents I talked to enforced plans like that in order to coordinate their various obligations and multiple responsibilities, their own feeding and their children's eating practices.

Even though mothers, and in some of the families fathers, are the main gatekeepers, their decisions are to a large extent influenced by children. Parents do the shopping and plan the meals with their children in mind (see Cook 2009). 11-year-old Kamila told me: "My mum buys only things that I will eat. It's not that she'll buy whatever I want, no, but in general she chooses things I like." Parents think about what their children have eaten last week or this week, and therefore what they would enjoy in the near future. They check what their children eat in school, to not repeat it at home. They try to predict when children will be hungry, and plan meals in such a way to adapt to children's needs. In many homes in Warsaw children non-intentionally affect the family foodways, and often dictate the family menus. But children are also often very intentional in their influences. In some families children are given a choice in what to eat. 43-year-old Paweł told me: "I usually ask them. I check what we have, and then let them decide what we eat from a couple of options I give them." Moreover, children often request particular dishes from the family menu. They also suggest new dishes, which they have tried elsewhere. 37-year-old Aneta's older son for example suggested a chicken baked with apples and plums which he had tried at his friend's home, and this meal has entered the family menu.

Thus feeding practices are often dictated by eating practices, as parents regularly, albeit reluctantly, give in to their children's wants:

> We try to be liberal in the boundaries and limits we set up, to adjust to them, talk with them, and give them what they like, what they are in a mood for (...) I have already learned what they don't eat, and I try to avoid these things, because this was a suicide – preparing something for half a day so that they don't even touch it.
> (Weronika, 30-year-old)

Parents employ diverse strategies which help them in organising the feeding process and implementing their ideas about what would be "proper".

However, they often have to adjust their ideas about feeding to the reality of children's tactics and practices, to their ideas, not necessarily reflexive or verbalized, about eating.

Family meals

Children shape the process of feeding in its many aspects and in many ways, during planning, shopping, preparing food and in the process of eating it. For example in most of the families from my research, not only the food that is eaten, but also the time of the dinner was adjusted to children's school and other time schedules. I direct my focus here to meals. As Mary Douglas explained, "each meal carries something of the meaning of the other meals; each meal is a structured social event which structures others in its own image" (1975, p. 240). Simultaneously, while being an element of a bigger structure, each of those food encounters is a dynamic event which involves various negotiations (see Boni 2016). Meals, Ochs and Shohet explain, are:

> Cultural sites where members of different generations and genders come to learn, reinforce, undermine, or transform each other's ways of acting, thinking, and feeling in the world, sometimes through cajoling, begging, probing, praising, bargaining, directing, ignoring, or otherwise interacting with one another in the course of nourishing one's body.
>
> (2006, p. 47)

Through these daily emotional interactions with food, children are cared for, but are also constantly controlled and governed. They respond to these controlling strategies in their own powerful, even if unintentional ways. Because of the changing family relations and the new position children have in many Polish families, today these responses seem to be manifested more visibly and more powerfully than they used to be a generation ago.

In order to feed their children in a way they want to, or to make sure that at least certain elements of their desired feeding are met, parents implement many strategies to which children respond with their own tactics. I discuss three of the most common.

Strategy 1: Eat at the table

Children should eat meals at the table. But it is often difficult to keep younger children sitting. They, intentionally or not, often disturb the organisation of feeding–eating situations. They do not want to eat, they get bored and they are distracted, they want to change seats, as Zuzia did. Or they want to break the rules. Children are not supposed to leave the table if adults do not excuse them.

I was told that this strategy of sitting children at the table, and keeping them there, is implemented for a couple of reasons. There is a practical component: children often make a mess when eating, so it is easier to clean it all up. But it is more than just about convenience; it is also what children should be taught, in a tautological way: meals are eaten at the table because it is a proper way to eat meals. Also, this allows parents to control children's food portions (see Anving and Thorsted 2010, p. 39). In fact, because of a need for that control, the parents I talked to usually did not allow children to put their own food on their own plates, as was the case with Bartek and Zuzia. Some parents told me how they love to eat dinner sitting on the couch in front of TV, but they rarely do this with their children as they need to show them examples of good behaviour, and one of the rules of the established adults' hegemonic order concerns eating at the table.

The strategy of sitting at the table while eating also entails teaching children table manners. A child needs to sit up straight, properly in the chair, and not for example laying on the table. She is supposed to eat with the cutlery, sometimes it is just a fork or a spoon. She should eat what is on the plate, and not eat from others' plates. The food should not be thrown. Mikołaj explained this to me:

> If I were to say that we constantly remind them to sit up straight, I would be lying; but if I said that we allow the complete chaos and running around the table, that would also not be true. Sadly, we are often tired and lose common sense, and they, because of their childish curiosity, they move around, something falls on the floor, sometimes it's funny and we joke about it, sometimes we use it as a starting point for a constructive remark, and sometimes we would just say "stop it!".

Children learn these social rules through constant repetition of disciplinary comments. When they are younger they resist it, and relate to diverse tactics, such as standing up, demanding to change seats, dancing around the table, eating with their hands, and taking food from other people's plates. They push the boundaries of the appropriate social behaviour to check how far they can take it and they exercise their powerful resistance to re-negotiate these rules. With time, they usually acknowledge that these are the social rules that need to be followed. They might even start reprimanding their younger siblings or their own toys if they do not behave properly at the table.

Strategy 2: Eat five more bites of meat and vegetables

Other strategies relate to what is eaten. Many parents referred to awful childhood memories, when they had to sit at the table until everything from their plate was eaten. It is quite striking that the generations of children brought up during the Polish People's Republic have so similar memories of being forced to eat. 32-year-old Kasia told me for example:

> There was a moment when he didn't eat meat at all. I did not worry about that. If he doesn't want it, he doesn't want it, I am not panicking. Sometimes it is annoying that I spend so much time preparing this, and he doesn't eat it, but I did not replace it with anything else. I remember how my parents yelled at me that I didn't eat; I do not want to repeat that. He eats as much as he wants. There is no such rule that he has to eat everything that is on the plate. He may finish it later.

Many parents told me that due to their memories, they do not want to force their children to eat. But they recognise how important it is that their children eat at least something from what they spent time preparing. Parents I talked to emphasize the importance of eating meals because of its nutritional value and a part of the social contract, rather than because of the pleasure food provides (see Ochs, Pontecorvo and Fasulo 1996). Preparing what children like usually solves this challenging issue. Family diets are planned with children in mind:

> I am not preparing things, which none of them likes; this is just not worth it! There are some things to which she would say that it is disgusting and she wouldn't eat it (...) I manage sometimes to do something more, so for example both the mielone [larger meatballs] and the chicken breast cutlets, if I have more time, but that happens rarely.
> (Magda, 40-year-old)

Magda, having three children and working three jobs, can rarely prepare something separate for each of them, so she has a food routine, a set menu for each week; so that each of her children can eat something they like every couple of days. Many parents talked about that kind of menu, an offer or repertoire of foods – from their point of view very limited – which is prepared for their children. Sometimes mothers would prepare something completely different for their children, as 30-year-old Marysia:

> I frequently indulge her. I allow her to eat whatever she wants. If she doesn't want to eat dinner, because there are vegetables, I am able to stand up from the table and cook something just for her. Because she is so stubborn, when she doesn't want to eat something she won't eat it. If I tell her that she has to eat it, she will not eat for the rest of the day, and I feel sorry for her.

Based on their study in Sweden, Anving and Sellerberg explain that parallel meals are often treated as something wrong, making them is a form of resignation or necessary submission, but they are prepared because children would not eat otherwise (2010, p. 206). This is a good example of their powerful and tactful influences over the process of feeding.

By not forcing children to eat, parents put themselves in a difficult position, as at the same time they want their children to eat what they "need" and to eat "properly". This causes a lot of anxiety, as expressed by Paulina:

> I know that people have diverse strategies, and some force their children to eat, sadly I sometimes do this as well. It is in the maternal instinct: this need to feed! And there is a scene sometimes because he has not finished his meal. Sometimes I'm mad at myself, how could I have led to such a situation that I force him to eat! But it is difficult when I think that he prefers to eat just bread rolls and apples, and he would be perfectly happy eating just that all the time. Not to mention the fact that I have cooked that soup or a delicious cutlet, and he sees one vein and does not want to eat it (…) then I enforce the strategy of ten – fifteen spoons, and he eats it. But this is not how I would like it to be!

At the table, there often is a need for flexibility and encouragement strategies. Parents usually do not force feed their children, but they use diverse strategies to persuade them to eat (see Paugh and Izquierdo 2009). The most common include such phrases as: "eat just five more spoons of soup and you will be done"; "eat just a small part of your meat and vegetables." Children are often "tricked" into eating vegetables; when they are grated finely, put into *pierogi* (dumplings) or whizzed in a soup, they cannot recognise them or pick them out. Parents also indicate on children's plates what should be eaten:

> It is not about her eating absolutely everything, we set the border: either on the plate, or in the amount of spoons or bites she needs to eat, it all depends on the likelihood of success.
>
> (Piotr, 35-year-old)

A child dictates this "likelihood of success" at a particular time and situation. Parents have to balance between what would satisfy them: how much food and what food ingredients are enough to count as a proper meal; their feeling that their child has eaten enough, with the probability that she will in fact eat it. And children do the same when deciding on eating more or refusing to eat. They learn to recognise how far they can push their parents on a certain occasion and how to negotiate, proposing to eat something that would satisfy their parents (e.g. vegetables), while avoiding eating something they do not want to eat (e.g. meat).

Another strategy is to offer dessert as a reward for complying with a parent's decision. Similarly, the refusal of dessert is treated as a way of persuading children to eat. As Piotr told me: "Usually we would not move to the next stage: the dessert." Conditional promises and negotiations are one way of persuading children, parents also use emotional pressure, as expressed by 36-year-old Asia:

> If she doesn't want to eat I will coax her, and tell her how it was when my parents worked in the field, and if my grandmother was not around, there was no dinner at all! I tell them they would understand and see how it is, if I stop cooking for a week!

Parents are obligated to feed their children. Children expect that they will be cared for and fed by their parents, and taking that expectation away, threatening to deliberately fail in fulfilling that obligation becomes one of the ways to persuade children to appreciate that they are fed and cared for, and encouraging them to eat.

While many parents in Warsaw restrain from force feeding their children and telling them that they have to sit at the table until everything from their plate is eaten, which was something they often experienced in their childhoods; when encouraging their children to eat they often relate to strategies similar to what their parents used in their childhoods. I, and many of my adult interlocutors, have heard in our childhoods stories about African children who are starving and about our parents' horrible memories from their childhoods of food scarcity. Children today hear something a bit different, and yet incredibly similar stories which also appeal to their sense of morality and guilt. The cycle will close, when in the future they will tell analogous stories to their own children in persuading them to eat.

Children use diverse verbal and non-verbal tactics to avoid eating what they do not want to eat or not in the way they are supposed to eat. Children's tactics include bluntly refusing to eat, pursing their lips, whining, tossing food to somebody else's plate or throwing it on the floor, crying. They also play one parent against each other, complain to one parent that they do not want to eat and the other parent is forcing them. They stall in hopes that adults will give up before they do. They are more or less successful in their tactics, as expressed by 11-year-old Krzysiek, Paulina's son: "If I like it, I will eat everything [and if not?] then I will not. My mum complains, but I always manage to leave something." During the meal children have to know how far they can push their parents and the boundaries that they set up, whether they can refuse to eat or should they eat just a little bit more. They tactfully resist parental feeding practices with their own non-eating practices.

Strategy 3: At least try it!

Another strategy relates to widening children's food horizons and encouraging them to try new things. Many parents attempt to persuade their children to at least try new foodstuffs, before dismissing them. James, Curtis and

Ellis discuss how children's refusal to try certain foods constitutes a symbolic refusal of participating in the family (2009, p. 45). They are encouraged to at least try because this makes them a part of the family. Anving and Sellerberg explain that next to *demarcation* through family meals (teaching children the family's own food culture), parents also attempt to "teach their children broad food tastes in the context of society at large (*diversity*) and to prepare the children for continuous change (*experimentation*)" (2010, p. 203). As 30-year-old Marysia explains:

> I attempt to persuade her to try. Sometimes we try saying "open your mouth, you will get a chocolate bar", but then she puts it in her mouth, and even before it is possible to taste anything, she spits it out.

Parents implement diverse strategies, such as promising a reward for complying with that rule, in order to persuade children to try new things. They are proud of children who are open to new tastes, and who develop a preference for more adult foods, such as herring, liver, spicier dishes. One of them even told me that "it means that children are open to new experiences in life."

During my research children often complained that parents force them to try new things. 12-year-old Agnieszka told me: "I don't like trying new things; I prefer to stick with what I know. And my parents torment me!" Children's tactics in avoiding to try new things mainly include refusing, trying to outwait their parents hoping that they will give up, taking food into their mouth and spitting it out right away, pretending that they tried, even if they did not, crying. They are usually successful in their tactics.

Conclusion

In this chapter I have discussed the strategies that parents employ in order to feed their children in a particular way, and children's responses with diverse tactics regarding eating (or non-eating). With that I argue for the relational approach to feeding and eating. Following Matthew Desmond (2014), I consider feeding and eating to be an interrelated process that involves various actors and spaces (though here limited to home and family). I focused on the boundaries, mental and physical, which parents and children build, bend and break when negotiating feeding and eating; and on the conflicts between them rather than their food culture. Such an analysis presents a very conflicted and antagonistic social world of family foodways. The conflicts and tensions, strategies and tactics resemble a battlefield more than anything else. And though this is how it often seemed to people I talked to, especially parents, they also talked about love, happiness and the practices of care connected with feeding their children. Similarly, for children, eating was both about struggles and about happy family moments and individual pleasures. Nevertheless, employing de Certeau's theory of strategies and tactics to family foodways allows us to see these power struggles in a new light.

This cycle of power, of adults' feeding strategies and children's tactics regarding eating, repeats itself in every generation. To some extent parents today reproduce what their parents have done, they sometimes unconsciously repeat particular strategies and very reflexively refrain from others; and children's behaviour resembles their parents' in their childhoods. However, new meanings and aspirations are attached to food and feeding children in Poland today, and the role of children has changed, giving them space for more powerful claims on their own eating. Because of diverse social, cultural and economic changes, related to family life, the notions of parenthood and childhood, and the food industry, the negotiations related to feeding and eating take significantly different forms today than they used to a generation ago. Back then the food choices were rather limited by external realities, while now they need to be limited by self-governing individuals, which puts great pressure on families (see Boni 2016).

Approaching feeding and eating through the relational lens enables us to look not only at individual practices and preferences regarding food, but rather consider them to be a part of the web of relationships and social entanglements. Mothers do not feed and children do not eat in a social vacuum. They are not only influenced by many other social actors, but also influence each other and shape each other's practices. Moreover, such an approach positions children as knowledgeable and skilful participants of social interactions. After all, both adults and children contribute to and make the feeding–eating relationships.

References

Abbots, E-J. and Lavis, A. (eds.) (2013) "Introduction. Contours of Eating: Mapping the Terrain of Body/Food Encounters" in *Why We Eat, How We Eat: Contemporary Encounters Between Foods and Bodies*. Farnham, Burlington: Ashgate. 1–14.

Anving, T. and Sellerberg, A.M. (2010) "Family Meals and Parent's Challenges". *Food, Culture and Society*, 13(2): 201–214.

Anving, T. and Thorsted, S. (2010) "Feeding ideals and the Work of Feeding in Swedish Families: Interactions of Mothers and Children Around the Dinner Table". *Food, Culture and Society*, 13(1): 29–46.

Boni, Z. (2015) "Negotiating Children's Food Culture in Post-socialist Poland". *Anthropology of Food*, Special Issue on Children's Food Heritage. Available from: https://aof.revues.org/7782.

Boni, Z. (2016) *Children and Food in Warsaw: Negotiating Feeding and Eating*. Unpublished PhD Thesis, Department of Anthropology and Sociology, SOAS: University of London.

Bourdieu, P. (1984) *Distinction: A Social Critique of the Judgement of Taste*. Trans. by Richard Nice. London: Routledge and Keegan Paul.

Cairns, K., and Johnston, J. (2015) *Food and Femininity*. London, New York: Bloomsbury Academic.
Charles, N., and Kerr, M. (1988) *Women, Food and Families*. Manchester: Manchester University Press.
Christensen, P. and James, A. (eds.) (2008) *Research with Children: Perspectives and Practices*. 2nd edition. Oxon, New York: Routledge.
Cook, D. (2009) "Children's Subjectivities and Commercial Meaning: The Delicate Battle Mothers Wage when Feeding their Children" in James, A., Kjørholt, A.T. & Tingstad, V. (eds.) *Children, Food and Identity in Everyday Life*. Basingstoke: Palgrave Macmillan. 112–129.
De Certeau, M. (1980) "On the Oppositional Practices of the Everyday Life". Trans. Frederic Jameson and Carl Lovitt. *Social Text* 3: 3–43.
De Certeau, M. (1984) *The Practice of Everyday Life*. Trans. Steven Rendall. Berkeley, London: University of California Press.
Desmond, M. (2014) "Relational Ethnography". *Theory and Society*, 43: 547–579.
DeVault, M. (1991) *Feeding the Family. The Social Organization of Caring as Gendered Work*. Chicago, London: University of Chicago Press.
Douglas, M. (ed) (1975) "Deciphering a Meal" in *Implicit Meanings: Essays in Anthropology*. London: Routledge. 36–54.
Giard, L. (1998) "Doing-Cooking" in de Certeau, M. *The Practice of Everyday Life. Volume 2: Living and Cooking*. London: University of Minnesota Press. 149–249.
Grieshaber, S. (1997) "Mealtime Rituals: Power and Resistance in the Construction of Mealtime Rules". *The British Journal of Sociology*, 48(4): 649–666.
Hays, S. (1996) *The Cultural Contradictions of Motherhood*. New Haven, CT: Yale University Press.
Hryciuk, R., Korolczuk, E. (eds.) (2012) *Pożegnanie z Matką Polką? Dyskursy, praktyki i reprezentacje macierzyństwa we współczesnej Polsce*. [Farewell to the Polish-Mother? Discourses, Practices and Representations of Motherhood in Contemporary Poland.] Warsaw: University of Warsaw Press.
James, A. and Curtis, P. (2010) "Family displays and personal lives". *Sociology*, 44(6): 1163–1180.
James, A., Curtis, P. and Ellis, K. (2009) "Negotiating Family, Negotiating Food: Children as Family Participants?" in James, A., Kjørholt, A.T. & Tingstad, V. (eds.) *Children, Food and Identity in Everyday Life*. Basingstoke: Palgrave Macmillan. 35–51.
James, A., Jenks, C. and Prout, A. (1998) *Theorizing Childhood*. Cambridge: Polity Press.
Lahire, B. (2011) *The Plural Actor*. Cambridge: Polity Press.
Mayall, B. (ed.) (1994) *Children's Childhoods: Observed and Experienced*. London: Falmer Press.
Murcott, A. (1983) "It's a pleasure to cook for him: Food, Mealtimes and Gender in some South Wales Households" in Garmanikow, E., Purvis, J. (eds.) *The Public and the Private*. London: Heinemann. 78–90.
Murcott, A. (2000) "Is it Still a Pleasure to Cook for Him? Social Changes in the Household and the Family". *Journal of Consumer Studies & Home Economics*, 24(2): 78–84.
Ochs, E., Pontecorvo, C. and Fasulo, A. (1996) "Socializing Taste". *Ethnos: Journal of Anthropology*, 61(1–2): 7–46.

Ochs, E. and Shohet, M. (2006) "The Cultural Structuring of Mealtime Socialization". *New Directions for Child and Adolescent Development*, Special Issue: Family Mealtime as a Context of Development and Socialization, 111: 35–49.

O'Connell, R. and Brannen, J. (2014) "Children's Food, Power and Control: Negotiations in Families with Younger Children in England". *Childhood*, 21(1): 87–102.

Ortner, S. (2006) *Anthropology and Social Theory*. Durham, NC and London: Duke University Press.

Paugh, A. and Izquierdo, C. (2009) "Why is There a Battle Every Night?: Negotiating Food and Eating in American Dinnertime Interaction". *Journal of Linguistic Anthropology*, 19(2): 185–204.

Strathern, M. (2012) "Eating (and Feeding)". *Cambridge Anthropology*, 30(2): 1–14.

Chapter 8

Feeding in context
Eating occasions as domestic socialized practice

David Marshall

> (T)he food practices that take place around the production and consumption of the family meal are also the medium through which processes of social identification take place on an everyday basis.
>
> (James et al. 2009: 49)

Socialisation and 'becomings'

Socialization is generally regarded as the process whereby individuals, through interactions with others, acquire specific skills, knowledge and behaviours that permit them to participate as members of a specific group or community (Dotson and Hyatt, 2005; John, 1999; Ward, 1974; Zigler and Child, 1969). The classic view is that children learn to 'become' consumers acquiring skills, social roles and associated behaviour that may form the basis of subsequent behaviour later in adulthood (Ward, 1974). Consequently, childhood is often seen as a 'work-in-progress' and socialization a one-way process – adult to child – where children learn, or are taught, how to behave in ways that will permit them to function as 'adult' consumers. This information – processing model of the young consumer adopts a Piagentian perspective and presents this as a linear process linked to cognitive development and experience although it is much more subtle than this and may be highly variable depending on the family context (Kerrane and Hogg, 2013; Epp and Price, 2008; John 1999). Parents play a key role in this socialization process (Cotte and Wood, 2004; Caruana and Vassallo, 2003; Carlson et al., 2001) although this influence will vary across age, class, children's participation and family type (McIntosh et al., 2010; Olsen and Ruiz, 2008; Neumark-Sztainer, et al., 2003, Moschis, 2001).

Children, for the most part, are regarded as 'incomplete' or 'becomings' (Qvortrup, 2004; James and Prout, 1990; James et al., 1998) – vulnerable to the market place pressures, less competent and lacking (economic) agency, in need of protection, often relying on parents to approve purchases and oversee their needs – in the transition to adulthood. The 'becoming' child is seen as an adult in the making (Johanssson, 2011). In conceptualizing this idea of 'becoming' we need to distinguish between 'becoming-the-same' thereby establishing and territorializing the existing order as in the socialization position and 'becoming-other' thereby escaping the existing order and de-territorializing through 'lines of flight' from the 'adult-in-charge' (Johansson, 2011; Deleuze and Guattari, 1984). These 'lines of flight' present opportunities for something new and different, to 'become-other', manifest as challenges to the existing order (Johansson, 2014), as exemplified by children challenging or questioning what they are expected to eat at family mealtimes (Ochs and Beck, 2013).

Whereas 'becoming-the-same' supports the existing order as children 'learn' to be (adult) consumers we have the alternative view of children as competent 'beings' with some agency and liberated from parental control (Johansson, 2011, 2006; Buckingham, 2011; Cook, 2009; James et al., 2009; Alanen, 1992; James and Prout, 1990; James et al., 1998; Qvortrup, 1987). Although this concept of 'being' celebrates children's resourcefulness and competencies it brings with it a 'burden of responsibility and separateness' (Aitken, 2008). However, it is not clear cut. As Johansson notes 'sometimes children appear as vulnerable "becomings" in need of protection and guidance and sometimes as competent beings with the capability to successfully navigate in consumer society' (Johansson, 2006: 332). There is a call to consider what lies in between the two extremes (Prout, 2005) and this is prevalent in the debates around the marketing of food to children where the evidence suggests a position somewhere between a compromised 'becoming' and a competent 'being' (Kline, 2011). The idea that all 'being' is in a permanent state of transition rather than a stable end point (Colebrook, 2002; Lee, 2001) does not negate the importance of capturing children's perspectives and consumption experiences in the moment. Moreover, children appear to have greater influence on family food decisions (Nørgaard and Brunsø, 2011; Nørgaard et al., 2007) with some evidence of reverse socialization and co-construction (Ayadi and Bree, 2010; Bugge and Almas, 2006; Cook, 2009; Ekström, 2007; Kerrane et al., 2012). The family meal is one of the many foodscapes children have to negotiate in their food socialisation (Brembeck et al., 2013).

Family mealtimes as social practice

The changing nature of the family and diversity of family life is reflected in the accounts of family food practices or 'doing family' (Jackson, 2009; Morgan, 1996, Warde, 2016). Individuals and groups confirm their family relationships through actions that are rooted in the everyday routines that emphasise the social nature of family practices and act as a conduit for shared meaning and identity (Finch, 2007). This is reflected in the conventional nature of mealtimes and as Ochs and Shohet note '[Mealtimes] ... are more or less conventional and demarcated as a kind of social practice that requires certain sensibilities of participants' (Ochs and Shohet, 2006: 36). These conventions can be seen in the 'eating scripts' that help us negotiate meals according to the time, the place and the participants (Douglas, 1972; Kjaernes et al., 2001; Marshall, 2005; Warde, 1997, Yates and Warde, 2016). In the case of families 'the proper dinner has retained its iconic status as a symbol for what a proper family does and is something that families aspire to' (James et al., 2009: 39). The 'family meal', 'proper meal', or 'hot "cooked dinner"', has become synonymous with British family life (Charles and Kerr, 1988; DeVault, 1991; Kemmer et al., 1998; Murcott, 1982; Grieshaber, 1997; Lupton, 1996; Marshall and Anderson, 2002; Ochs and Shohet, 2006; O'Connell and Brannen, 2014; Valentine, 1999). It can be seen elsewhere in the 'food ideal', i.e. the informal norm of what and with who to eat that informs food related decisions, particularly for households with children (Holttinen, 2014). The family meal offers an opportunity to consider the practices of children at the domestic table (Ochs and Shohet, 2006). Whereas mealtime rituals serve as a regulatory mechanism to discipline and 'normalise' (Greishaber, 1997), children appear capable of making independent choices that can lead to (re)negotiation over household consumption practices (Cook, 2009; James et al., 2009; James and Curtis, 2010; Valentine, 1999). These practices involve demanding, taking and refusing food as parents overtly, or covertly, encourage or restrict consumption of particular foods (see Boni, this volume). This results in different patterns of negotiation and control of food that include resistance, hierarchical, negotiated and child control (O'Connell and Brannen, 2014).

Demarcation and synchronisation of taste

The family meal forms an important part of the child's integration into the family unit in what Anving and Sellerberg (2010) term 'demarcation'. In this process children are socialised into family eating habits in order to align their tastes with family preferences and integrate them into the family way of eating, avoiding the need to prepare 'parallel' meals. But this is not simply a one-way process, as Anving and Sellerberg comment '(F)ood-mediated socialization is an intensive, direct process that calls for active participation of the child; it is not simply that the child is shown what is right' (2010: 204). There appears to be sufficient flexibility around this integration into family life to allow children to experiment with new foods and tastes. This can be seen more broadly in a trend towards more variety in family meals and new ideas about what constitutes proper meals or what dishes can be included (Beardsworth and Keil, 1997; Blake et al., 2009; Marshall and Pettinger, 2009). Moreover, new dishes may be introduced to the family by the children, echoing Ekström's (2007) idea of reverse socialisation and different dishes may be prepared in some households to accommodate children's preferences (Ochs and Beck, 2013). Brembeck (2009), reporting on immigrant Swedish families, argues that the family meal is where children learn to restrict their own tastes and desires and learn 'family tastes'. As she says (after Sellerberg 2008),

> the synchronisation of tastes is very much what children do. Where it is normally considered that the children are the ones who are supposed to change – to restrict childish or egotistical tastes and mature to appreciate the broader range of healthy foods that are considered socially acceptable and 'normal' – in frontier families this synchronisation is to a large extent in the hands of the children.
> (Brembeck, 2009: 139)

In complying with and accepting these cultural norms children are 'becoming-the-same'.

Pressures on the family meal

Families continue to eat together in spite of increasing demands on their time due to work and school commitments (Brannen et al., 2013; Cappellini and Parsons, 2012; Cheng et al., 2007; L'huissier et al., 2013; Marshall and Pettinger, 2009; Meiselman, 2009; Ochs and Beck, 2013). Most family meals take place at home and children see these as important eating events they are expected to participate in (Burke et al., 2007; Fulkerson et al., 2006; Haapalahti et al., 2003; McIntosh et al., 2009).

Parents face the challenge of providing a nutritional diet while accommodating individual likes and dislikes and trying to satisfy all the family preferences in one meal (Hughner and Maher, 2006). Older children (10–13 years old) appear generally satisfied with family food and have most influence on small meals such as breakfast, lunch, and snacks with less influence on the more labour-intensive family dinner (Nørgaard et al., 2007; Warren et al., 2008). This influence extends to where to eat (meal locations) and when to eat (meal times). Where the meal is eaten often depends on the configuration of the domestic space but the decision to watch television during meals may see the meal relocate from the kitchen or dining room to the lounge or the child's bedroom (Chitakunye and Maclaran, 2014; Fitzpatrick et al., 2007). In low income families, space restrictions and economic constraints mean that sitting at a dining table remains an aspiration. Although dinners were usually eaten in front of the television, eating together as a family remains important (Harden, 2013). Meal times may be relocated to accommodate work and leisure activities of different family members or fit in with other schedules. Breakfast and lunch are more likely to be eaten alone or outside of the family home unit whereas evening meals are shared with the family (Sobal and Nelson, 2003).

Family meals provide an opportunity to bring the nuclear family together and create a sense of unity but they are also a potential site for conflict (Lupton, 1996; Ochs and Beck, 2013) and children may resist parental attempts to get them to eat proper meals or consume healthy foods. The solution is a compromise and 'usually consists of a family agreement on a combination of "proper meals" all together and alternative, separated meals for parents and children reflecting their tastes' (Romani, 2005: 251). Meals clearly play an important role in children's food socialization and this chapter looks at how children engage in that consumption experience.

Research methods

This qualitative study looked at food experiences of children aged between 8 and 11. At this age food preferences and tastes are developing and children are able to think more conceptually, to categorize and discuss their own experiences and ideas about who they are (Chaplin and John, 2005; John, 1999). Moreover, they are exposed to eating both inside and outside the home and are not completely reliant on their parents for all their food choices. Research questions were broad ranging but included questions about their meals, snacking and favourite foods.

Given the exploratory nature of the research, discussion groups were used as an appropriate interpretive research method allowing us to reveal the issues that were relevant to the children themselves (Gunter and Furnham, 1998; Lawlor and Prothero, 2011; Moore and Lutz, 2000). Head teachers were approached at two primary schools in a major UK city. Due to the challenges of recruiting and gaining access to schools this was a convenience sample and both schools are situated in predominantly middle class catchment areas of the city. Permission to talk to the children was granted by the head teacher who approved this with the classroom teachers and parents. Each parent was sent a letter describing the research project and requesting permission for the children to take part. Further permission was requested from the relevant authorities. All children had the option to opt out of the research. Children were provided with information in advance of the research and debriefed after the project.

A total of eight discussion groups were carried out at two schools in the same catchment area. The first school visits took place in May 2006. Two focus groups were conducted with Primary 4 children (aged 8 and 9 years old) and two with Primary 6 children (aged 10 and 11 years old). The second school visits were carried out in November and December 2006. Two discussion groups were conducted with Primary 5 children (aged 9 years old) and Primary 6 (aged 10 years old). All the groups contained both boys and girls and were conducted in the classroom with the teacher present but situated away from the group. Focus groups were moderated by the author and each child who was a member of the class had the opportunity to participate. A total of 106 children participated in the focus groups with a mode of thirteen children and a maximum of fifteen children in any one classroom group. As the sessions were classroom based, and access to the schools centred on in-classroom activities, it was felt important to be inclusive although this resulted in larger numbers in the discussion groups. Although smaller groups might have been desirable there were also practical considerations around the classroom time available and a need to minimise disruption to the teaching activities. While small groups of young children do not always generate spontaneous debate the main challenge in conducting the groups was ensuring that everyone had an opportunity to speak when there were dominant voices in the groups. As the children all knew each other they were 'not shy in coming forward' and offering their views although most children adopted a classroom approach and raised their hands when they wanted to talk which facilitated the discussion. The children appeared comfortable with this. As the groups progressed some children contributed to the discussion without raising their hands or asking permission. One of the main challenges was in 'managing' the discussion as there was a tendency for sub-groups to form and talk about the issues raised.

Groups were audio recorded and children were informed that everything they said was confidential and would not be attributed to them as individuals. All of the focus groups were transcribed verbatim and the transcripts analysed for emerging issues and themes both within groups and across groups (Spiggle, 1994). The transcriptions consisted of 136 pages of text and formed the basis for the data analysis that involved listening to the interviews, reading and annotating the transcripts to identify key issues and emergent themes. Initial findings were presented to one of the schools for feedback and comment.

Findings

Children's accounts show how their ideas about meals are framed in relation to other eating events and how they identify with and relate to these events.

Family meals as practice

The discussion centred on meals eaten at home with parents and siblings; there were relatively few references to eating outside the home. Children clearly understood the eating scripts they had been exposed to and were able to draw a number of distinctions between meals and snacks (Curtis et al., 2010) reflecting learned social conventions surrounding these two types of eating event. For example, meals were restricted to the beginning, middle and end of the day, they were usually eaten hot, served on a plate and required the eater to sit down at the table or occasionally in front of the television. Children understood the routines and rituals of family meals as well as what foods are associated with family meals and 'proper' eating (as opposed to snacks) (Lupton, 1996; Marshall, 2005). They talked about meals in relation to their experiences of eating dinner at home with the family (Burke et al., 2007; Haapalahti et al., 2003; McIntosh et al., 2009). A number of children referred to their main meal as 'tea', and on these occasions the children were expected to 'sit down' at the table and use cutlery, in part due to the practicalities of eating (usually hot) food off a plate. However, the distinction between meals and snacks was not always clear cut, for example, while meals were usually 'hot' and 'cooked' one of the children talked about eating cold pizza, another about having cold fish and chips. Some foods, like ice cream, could be eaten as a main meal desert or a snack; in the first case signalling the end of the meal in the second being served as a treat. It is these subtleties in practice that children learn in the process of their food socialization and in 'becoming-the-same'. Meals eaten at home provide an opportunity to learn the rules and an environment in which identity is performed. It is the family evening meal, or dinner, that is seen as the main occasion revered for eating together and associated with eating 'properly'; regardless of how often it occurs in practice. This is one of the few occasions when families get together (Ochs and Beck, 2013) and for these children meals were strongly linked to 'doing family'.

Becoming-the-same: the serious matter of family dinner

Accounts of family meals convey a sense of belonging, as part of the family, as in 'normally' having dinner with mum and dad, or with the extended family, as in eating traditional roast dinner at grandmother's house thus enacting the 'food ideal' (Holttinen, 2014; Mosio et al., 2004). As increased pressure on family time creates challenges for all the family to sit down together these family meals take on even more importance, materially and symbolically. Participation, or taking part, is the key and although the children may have few alternatives at this age they do not appear to be resentful of the family meal but engage with it.

The family meal is an opportunity for children to spend time with other family members. This allows them to establish their collective identity by participating in the meal as members of the family and, at the same time, express individual preferences through eating specific dishes and or requesting favourite foods. There was no discussion in the groups about resistance to family meals, either in terms of refusing the food (as with younger children) or refusing to participate in the meal. This is more suggestive of demarcation and 'becoming-the-same' (Johansson, 2011) as children conform to their parent's wishes (O'Connell and Brannen, 2014). That is not to say there is always agreement but these children felt that they had some influence on what they ate at the family meal.

Individual likes and dislikes are accommodated within the family meal repertoire with specific preferences permitted in minor courses or in the choice (or not) of vegetables. The main components or the staples are less likely to be subject to negotiation. In some households children are permitted to choose their dessert (pudding) course having eaten their main meal. Involving children in the meal preparation can lead to healthier diets (van der Horst et al., 2014) but few of these children helped prepare family meals which is consistent with research in American households (Ochs and Beck, 2013). Almost all the children said that it was their mother who prepared dinner and there was little discussion of fathers or children preparing food (DeVault, 1991; Murcott, 1982).

Becoming other and being: relaxing the rules

Children readily accepted, and bought into, the idea of eating family meals as an important part of 'family life' or how they 'do' family. Most reported eating the same meals as their parents and proffered a wide range of favourite dishes from traditional roast dinners through to takeaway meals that clearly reflected their exposure to a relatively broad cuisine. Pizza and pasta dishes such as spaghetti bolognaise and lasagne were cited as regular family meals appearing once a week or more frequently. Other favourites included fish/seafood, meat dishes (lamb, steak, steak pie, roast dinners, roast beef with gravy and Yorkshire puddings), fried potato chips, Chinese (lemon chicken, chicken fried rice, duck dumplings) and Indian (chicken curry) dishes. While we do not know if these choices are instigated by children or their parents it supports the idea of 'menu pluralism' (Beardsworth and Keil, 1997) reflecting some of the meal variation and variety that other researchers have found. What we see is a wider range of favourites dishes, and cuisines, beyond the more traditional 'meat and two veg' traditionally associated with the 'proper' family dinner; although favourite dishes are not necessarily reflective of what children eat on a daily basis.

This may be seen as evidence of children 'becoming' food consumers, accepting the foods and dishes associated with 'proper meals', although there are a number of 'lines of flight' that exist (Johansson, 2014). Individual preferences, for example steak, were not often part of the regular family meals but seen as an occasional or special treats. Other 'treats' included meals eaten out in a restaurant or takeaway meals eaten at home. Eating out at a restaurant was a special treat for most of these children whereas take away meals eaten at home were a more regular occurrence. These were seen as distinctly different from regular family meals both in terms of what was eaten and when they were permitted. Takeaway meals, such as bought in pizza, or Indian or Chinese dishes were usually weekend treats (for adults as well as children!). On these occasions the 'normal' rules about eating were often relaxed and the meal might be eaten away from the table, or without the usual cutlery. This informality was part of their appeal (see Caraher et al., 2004) and represented an opportunity for the family to spend time together in a more relaxed and informal setting engaged in other activities such as watching television (Chitakunye and Maclaran, 2014). With takeaway dinners children may be allowed to select the dishes or choose individual items in a way that is not always permissible, or practical, when sitting down to a home prepared dinner. The range and variety of dishes mentioned suggest that the family meal may be much less restrictive in terms of what is eaten reflecting more diversity and experimentation (Anving and Sellerberg, 2010; Marshall and Pettinger, 2009). On these less formal occasions we expect more 'becoming-other' or 'being', in terms of individual choices (Marshall, 2016).

Discussion

This chapter offers an insight into children's perspectives on food practices and the role that family meals play in their everyday food experiences. In addressing this gap in our knowledge the research contribution lies in a more nuanced understanding of how children relate to meals as part of their ongoing socialization and finds that rather than resisting family meals these children appear to be embracing family meals as part of 'doing' family. Moreover, whereas parents may ultimately decide what is served at the family meal (Ayadi and Bree, 2010) there was relatively little conflict in these accounts and children appeared to be both aware, and accepting, of the rules and rituals surrounding the family meal. The ideology and symbolic value of the family meal remains important and parental attempts to maintain a coherent family identity, through provision of 'proper meals', is punctuated by regular challenges and disruptions to this identity practice that are contained within specific parts of the family meal (see Webster, this volume). 'Lines of flight' range from negotiation around individual components of the meal to the opportunity to relax the rules and participate in less formal meals that are seen as fun and something the family can enjoy together. Negotiation between parents and children is part of everyday family food practice but rather than leading to conflict normative practice can accommodate both collective and individual identities, and reflect the range of experiences within families (Kerrane and Hogg, 2013).

Food socialization is often seen as a one way process, from parents to children, but there is little attempt to consider the mediating role of context on this process. Children are socialized into eating 'properly' and in participating in the family dinner are 'becoming same' (Figure 8.1). Opportunities to deviate from the eating script, choosing dessert or negotiating around their vegetables, offer 'lines of flight' allowing children to express individual likes and dislikes, but still sanctioned and approved by parents. Deviation from the rules is more acceptable in light meals and while this point of

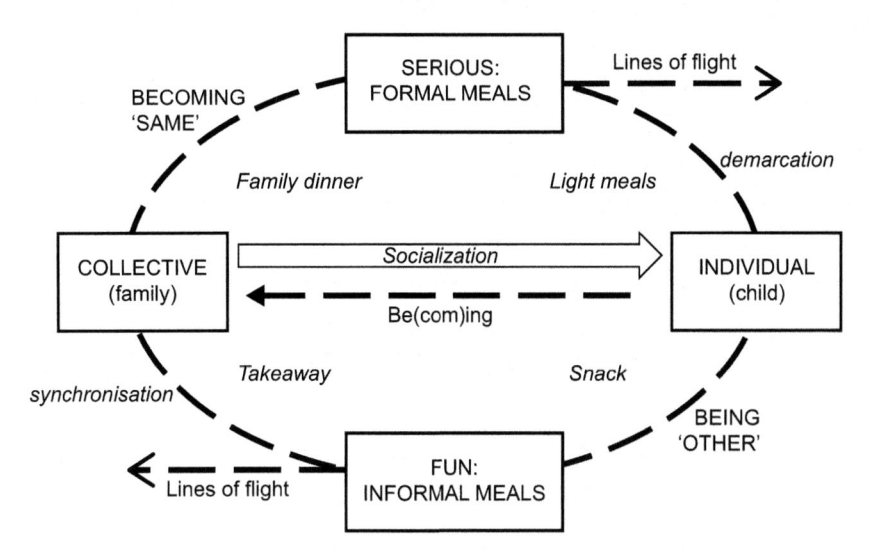

Figure 8.1 Family meals and identity practice

demarcation serves to challenge, rather than threaten the family meal, it permits more individualized eating that centers on the child and 'being other'. These less formal eating occasions involve small individual items such as snacks that do not threaten the meal but represent different practices (Marshall, 2016) and additional lines of flight. Takeaway dinners embody this idea of informality and fun where individuals can select what they want but they draw children back into synchronized family eating. Lines of flight (Deleuze and Guattari, 1984) provide flexibility and a release from the overly prescriptive and restrictive nature of the family dinner. Rather than seeing food socialization as a one-way process it is mediated by the nature of the occasion and children, through those experiences, are both simultaneously 'becoming same' and 'being other' food consumers. Children's experience of family meals are extremely diverse but in focusing on the food and the consumer, rather than the context, we fail to understand how and where food fits into family food consumption.

One could speculate that this commitment to the family meal may be a function of this age group (tweens), a feature of their upbringing (middle class), their limited awareness of covert influences, or even an inability or unwillingness to recall negative family meal experiences. However, it may also reflect the willingness of parents to respond directly to their children's meal requests or to respond indirectly by serving what they know their children like (and will eat). Individual preferences can be accommodated in specific courses (such as dessert), or on specific occasions (informal weekend takeaway dinners). Children appear to be willing to accept the normative practice of eating properly – 'becoming-the-same' – in exchange for an opportunity to influence what is served in specific parts of the meal system. These accounts support the idea that children have more influence on small meals and snacks rather than family dinners (Short, 2003; Norregaard et al., 2007) but there are 'lines-of-flight' within family meals that allow them to pursue individual identity projects alongside this collective eating activity.

Children are developing eating practices in context, selectively adapting their eating practices to different situations and in the process contributing to that foodscape. This suggests that children are both cognizant of, and compliant with, adapting their behavior to the situation and this, in turn, may allow them to employ their own identity projects elsewhere (Johansson, 2014, Marshall, 2010b). However, while eating meals is about identifying with the family there is a still a sense that, for many of these children, food has to be 'good to eat' as well as 'good to think' (Douglas, 1972). In this discussion around family meals there was little reference to specific food brands and an unspoken assumption that, with the exception of takeaways, the food was 'homemade' and fitted with the food ideal (Holttinen, 2014; Mosio et al., 2004). Understanding where and how specific products fit into that family meal practice has implications for how food products are promoted and positioned and adds to our understanding of food choice, and the implications in terms of product sales related to health and convenience (Carrigan and Szmigin, 2006; Marshall and Pettinger, 2009).

This study has a number of limitations. It is a small sample of middle class children in one geographical location so extrapolating the findings to other cultural or social contexts is not possible but it does provide some insights into the nature of children's socialisation as part of the family unit and their identity practice. The fact that the children all knew each other may limit the range of views and perspectives offered in the groups and the large numbers in the discussion groups limit the contribution for each child. Despite this the groups provided a familiar environment in which to encourage discussion and allowed the children to offer their perspectives on eating as part of the family.

Conclusions

It appears that young children are being socialised into eating properly and, to borrow from Johansson (2006), are more 'becoming' than 'being' when it comes to family meals. But children continue, by their presence at the table, to influence the nature and form of the family meal. Food remains an important part of family life and of children's collective identity. Rather than having their tastes subordinated to fit with the adult world of mealtimes children are allowed some autonomy, to such an extent that their preferences play a role in shaping family food choice (Cook, 2009).

The discourse around childhood socialization implies a one-way transmission from adults to children and one that presumes a relatively passive child. This research challenges that idea and views this process as more engaging of children through a form of 'co-creation' that involves some degree of reverse socialization (Ekström, 2007). Children contribute to and influence ideas about family meals, albeit bounded and constrained within certain parameters, and participating in the ritual of family meal adds to their sense of identity and provides an opportunity for 'doing' family. Furthermore, while much of children's food socialisation is about compliance, or 'becoming-the-same', there are a number of 'lines of flight', sanctioned by parents and facilitated by the food industry, that accommodate 'becoming-other'. Rather than seeing these as two opposing or conflicting states it may be that we are witnessing an emergent collective and individual identity that co-exists as 'be(com)ing' where individual identities are difficult to distinguish from collective identities as a consequence of the 'dynamic interplay' between them. Perhaps it is time to move beyond this simple dualistic model and begin to understand children as relational beings interacting and engaging with other family members and the marketplace (Epp and Price, 2008; Cook, 2009). Family identity is never coherent and children regularly punctuate parent's attempts to maintain a cohesive identity. To this extent we should encourage more research on children as a relatively underrepresented part of the family unit in order to understand the contribution they make to how we think about family meals.

References

Aitken, S. C. (2008) Desarrollo integral y fronteras/Integral development and borderscapes. In S. C. Aitken, R. Lund and A. T. Kjörhol, (eds.) *Global Childhoods: Globalization, Development and Young people*, London and Sage: Routledge.

Alanen, L. (1992) *Modern Childhood? Exploring the 'Child Question' in Sociology*. Institute for Educational Research. Publication series A, Research Report 50. Jyväskylä: University of Jyväskylä.

Anving, T. and Sellerberg, A. (2010) Family meals and parent's challenges, *Food, Culture and Society*, 13(2), 201–214.

Ayadi, K. and Bree, J. (2010) An ethnography of the transfer of food learning within the family, *Young Consumers*, 11(1), 67–76.

Beardsworth, A. and Keil, T. (1997) *Sociology on the Menu: An Invitation to the Study of Food and Society*. London: Routledge.

Blake, M., Mellor, J.Crane, L., and Osz, B. (2009) Eating in time, eating up time. In P. Jackson, (ed.) *Changing Families, Changing Food*. London: Palgrave Macmillan, 187–2014.

Brannen, J., O'Connell, R. and Mooney, A. (2013) Families, meals and synchronicity: eating together in British dual earner households, *Community, Work and Family*, 16 (4), 417–434.

Brembeck, H. (2009) Children's 'becoming' in frontiered foodscapes. In A. James, A. Kjørholt and V. Tingstad (eds.) *Children, Food and Identity in Everyday Life.* London: Palgrave Macmillan, 130–148.

Brembeck, H., Johansson, B., Bergström, K., Engelbrektsson, P., Hillén, S., Jonsson, L., Karlsson, A., Ossiansson, E., and Shanahan, H. (2013) Exploring children's foodscapes, *Children's Geographies*, 11(1), 74–88.

Buckingham, D. (2011) *The Material Child: Growing up in Consumer Culture*, Cambridge: Polity.

Bugge, A. B. and Almas, R. (2006) Domestic dinner: representations and practices of a proper meal among young suburban mothers, *Journal of Consumer Culture*, 6(2), 203–228.

Burke, S. J., McCarthy, S. N., O'Neill, J. L., Haannon, E. M., Kiely, M.Flynn, A. and Gibney, M. J. (2007) An examination of the influence of eating location on diets of Irish children, *Public Health Nutrition*, 10(6), 601–607.

Cappellini, B. and Parsons, E. (2012) Sharing the meal: food consumption and family identity. In R. Belk (ed.), *Research in Consumer Behaviour*, 14, 109–128.

Caraher, M., Baker, H. and Burns, M. (2004) Children's views of cooking and food preparation, *British Food Journal*, 106(4), 255–273.

Carlson, L., Laczniak, R. N. and Walsh, A. (2001), Socializing children about television: an intergenerational study, *Journal of the Academy of Marketing Science*, 29(3), 277–288.

Carrigan, M. and Szmigin, I. (2006) "Mothers of invention": maternal empowerment and convenience consumption, *European Journal of Marketing*, 40(9/10), 1122–1142.

Caruana, A. and Vassallo, R. (2003) Children's perception of their influence over purchases: the role of parental communication patterns, *Journal of Consumer Marketing*, 20(1), 55–66.

Chaplin, N. J. and John, D. R. (2005) The development of self-brand connections in children and adolescents, *Journal of Consumer Research*, 32 (June), 119–129.

Charles, N. and Kerr, M. (1988) *Women, Food and Families*. Manchester: Manchester University press.

Cheng S.L., OlsenW., Southerton, D. & WardeA. (2007) The changing practice of eating: evidence from UK time diaries, 1975 and 2000, *The British Journal of Sociology*, 58(1), 39–61.

Chitakunye, D. P. and Maclaran, P. (2014) Materiality and family consumption: the role of television in changing mealtime rituals, *Consumption, Markets and Culture*, 17(1), 50–70.

Colebrook, C. (2002) *Gilles Deleuze*. London: Routledge.

Cook, D. T. (2009) Semantic provisioning of children's food: commerce, care and maternal practice, *Childhood*, 16(3), 317–334.

Cotte, J. and Wood, S. L. (2004), Families and innovative consumer behaviour: a triadic analysis of sibling and parental influence, *Journal of Consumer Research*, 31, 78–86.

Curtis, P., James, A. and Ellis, K. (2010) Children's snacking, children's food: food moralities and family life, *Children's Geographies*, 8(3), 291–302.

Deleuze, G. and Guattari, F. (1984) *Anti-Oidipus: Capitalism and Schizophreniza*. London: Athlone.

DeVault, M. (1991) *Feeding the Family: The Social Organisation of Sharing as Gendered Work*. Chicago, IL: University of Chicago Press.

Dotson, M. J. & Hyatt, E. M. (2005). Major influence factors in children's consumer socialization, *Journal of Consumer Marketing*, 22(1), 35–42.

Douglas, M. (1972) Deciphering a Meal, *Dædalus*, 101(1), 61–81 (reprinted in Implicit Meanings: Essays in Anthropology, Routledge and Kegan Paul, London, 1975, 249–275).

Ekström, K. M. (2007) Parental consumer learning or 'keeping up with the children', *Journal of Consumer Behavior*, 6(4), 203–217.

Epp, A. M. & Price, L. L. (2008) Family identity: a framework of identity interplay in consumption practices, *Journal of Consumer Research*, 35, 50–70.

Finch, J. (2007) Displaying families, *Sociology*, 41(1), 65–81, DOI: doi:10.1177/0038038507072284.

Fitzpatrick, E., Edmunds, L. S. and Dennison, B. A. (2007) Positive effects of family meals undone by television viewing, *Journal of American Dietetic Association*, 107(4), 666–671.

Fjellström, C. (2009) The Family Meal in Europe. In H. Meiselman, (ed.) *Meals in Science and Practice: Interdisciplinary Research and Business Applications*. Oxford: Woodhead, 219–235.

Fulkerson, J. A., Neumark-Sztainer, D., Story, M. (2006) Adolescent and parent views of family meals, *Journal of American Dietetic Association*, 106(4), 527–532.

Grieshaber, S. (1997) Mealtime rituals. Power and resistance in the construction of mealtime rules, *British Journal of Sociology*, 48(4), 649–666.

Gunter, B. and Furnham, A. (1998) *Children as Consumers: A Psychological Analysis of the Young People's Market*. London: Routledge.

Haapalahti, M., Mykkänen, H., Tikkanen, S. and Kokkonen, J. (2003) Meal patterns and food use in 10–11-year-old Finnish Children. *Public Health Nutrition*, 6(4), 365–370. cited in Fjellström, C. (2009).

Harden, J. (2013) Food and finance: mothers' food practices with young children, on a low income, *Scottish School of Public Health*, Research Briefing 4, August 2013. http://ssphr.files.wordpress.com/2013/08/ssphr_briefing_4.pdf (accessed January 2017).

Holttinen, H. (2014) How practices inform the materialization of cultural ideals in mundane consumption, *Consumption Markets and Culture*, 17(6), 573–594.

Hughner, R. S. and Maher, J. K. (2006) Factors that influence parental food purchases for children: implications for dietary health, *Journal of Marketing Management*, 22(9/10), 929–954.

James, A. and Curtis, P. (2010) Family displays and personal lives, *Sociology*, 44(6), 1163–1180.

James, A. and Prout, A. (eds.) (1990) *Constructing and Reconstructing Childhood: Contemporary Issues in the Sociological Study of Childhood*. London: The Falmer Press.

James, A., Curtis, P. and Ellis, K. (2009) Negotiating family, negotiating food: children as family participants? In A. James, A. T. Kjørhold and V. Tingstad (eds.) *Children, Food and Identity in Everyday Life*. London: Palgrave Macmillan, 35–51.

James, A., Jenks, C., and Prout, A. (1998) *Theorising Childhood*. Oxford: Polity Press.

Jackson, P. (ed.) (2009). *Changing Families, Changing Food*. London: Palgrave Macmillan.

Johansson, B. (2006) Children and their money, *European Advances in Consumer Research*, 7, 327–332.

Johansson, B. (2011) Doing adulthood in childhood research, *Childhood*, 19(1), 101–114.

Johansson, B. (2014) Lines of flight in children's foodscapes. Paper presented at 6th International Child and Teen consumption conference, University of Edinburgh Business School.

John, D. R. (1999) Consumer socialization of children: a retrospective look at twenty-five years of research, *Journal of Consumer Research*, 26(3), 183–213.

Kemmer, D., Anderson, A. and Marshall, D. (1998) Living together and eating together: changes in food choice and eating habits during the transition to married/cohabiting, *The Sociological Review*, 46(1), 48–72.

Kerrane, K. B., Bettany, S. M. and Kerrane, K. (2015) Siblings as socialization agents: exploring the role of 'sibship' in the consumer socialization of children, *European Journal of Marketing*, 49(5/6), 713–735.

Kerrane, B. and Hogg, M. (2013) Shared or non-shared? Children's different consumer socialisation experiences within the family environment, *European Journal of Marketing*, 7(3/4), 506–524.

Kerrane, B., Hogg, M. and Bettany, S. M. (2012) Children's influence strategies in practice: exploring the co-constructed nature of the child influence process in family consumption, *Journal of Marketing Management*, 27(7/8), 809–835.

Kjaernes, U., Ekström, M. P., Gronow, J., Holm, L., & Mäkelä, J. (2001). Introduction. In U. Kjaernes, et al. (eds.) *Eating patterns. A day in the lives of nordic peoples*. Lysaker: SIFO-National Institute for Consumer Research, pp. 25–63.

Kline, S. (2011) *Globesity, Food Marketing and family Lifestyles*. Basingstoke: Palgrave MacMillan. doi:10.1177/0907568205051906

Lawlor, M. A. and Prothero, A. (2011) Pester power – a battle of wills between children and their parents, *Journal of Marketing Management*, 27(5/6), 561–581.

Lee, N. (2001) *Childhood and Society: Growing up in an Age of Uncertainty*. Buckingham and Philadelphia: Open University Press.

L'Hussier, A., Tichit, C., Caillavet, F., Cardon, P., Masullo, A.Martin-Fernandez, J., Parizot, I. and Chauvin, P. (2013) Who still eats three meals a day? Findings from a quantitative survey in the Paris area, *Appetite*, 63, 59–69.

Lupton, D. (1996) *Food, the Body and the Self*. London: Sage.

McIntosh, W. A., Dean, W., Torres, C. C., Anding, J., Kubena, K. S. and Naya, R. (2009) The American family meal. In H. Meiselman, (ed.) *Meals in Science and Practice: Interdisciplinary Research and Business Applications*, Oxford: Woodhead, 190–218.

McIntosh, W. A., Kubena, K. S., Tolle, G. W. R.Jie-sheng , J. and Anding, J. (2010) Mothers and meals: the effects of mothers' meal planning and shopping motivations on children's participation in family meals, *Appetite*, 55(3), 623–628.

Marshall, D. (2005) Food as ritual, routine or convention. *Consumption, Markets and Culture*, 8(1), 69–85.

Marshall, D. (2010a) (ed.) *Understanding Children as Consumers*. London: Sage.

Marshall, D. (2010b) Be(com)ing consumers: young children's everyday accounts of snacking, Special Session: The Family that eats together {.} : Food Discourses that shape the Consuming family. *European Association of Consumer Research*, Royal Holloway University of London, Surrey, UK, June 30th to July 3rd.

Marshall, D. (2016) Meal deviations: children's food socialisation and the practice of snacking. In B. Cappellini, D. Marshall and L. Parsons (eds.) *The Marketisation of the Meal: Marketplace Practices, Discourses and Consumers*. London: Routledge.

Marshall, D. and Anderson, A. (2002) Proper meals in transition: young married couples on the nature of eating together, *Appetite*, 39, 193–206.

Marshall, D. and Pettinger, C. (2009) Revisiting British Meals. In H. Meiselman, (ed.) *Meals in Science and Practice: Interdisciplinary Research and Business Applications.* Oxford: Woodhead, 638–664.

Meiselman, H. (2009) *Meals in Science and Practice: Interdisciplinary Research and Business Applications.* Oxford: Woodhead.

Moore, E. S. and Lutz, R. J. (2000) Children, advertising and product experiences: a multimethod inquiry, *Journal of Consumer Research*, 27(1), 31–48.

Morgan, D. H. J. (1996), *Family Connections: An Introduction to Family Studies.* Cambridge, MA: Blackwell.

Moschis, G. (2001) The role of family communication in the socialization of adolescents and children, *Journal of Consumer Research*, 11, March, 898–913.

Mosio, R., Arnould, E. J. and Price, L. L. (2004) Between mothers and markets: constructing family identity through homemade food, 4(3), 361–384.

Murcott, A. (1982) On the social significance of the 'cooked dinner' in South Wales, *Social Science Information*, 21(4/5), 677–695.

Neumark-Sztainer, D., Hannan, P. J., Story, M., Croll, J., & Perry, C. (2003). Family meal patterns. Associations with sociodemographic characteristics and improved dietary intake among adolescents, *Journal of the American Dietetic Association*, 103, 317–322.

Nørgaard, M. K., and Brunsø, K. (2011) Family conflicts regarding food choices, *Journal of Consumer Behaviour*, 10(3), 141–151.

Nørgaard, M., Kümpel, K., Bruns, P., Harudrup, C. and Romero Mikkelsen, R. (2007) Children's influence on and participation in the family decision process during food buying, *Young Consumers*, 8(3), 197–216.

O'Connell, R. and Brannen, J. (2014) Children's food, power and control: negotiations in families with younger children in England. *Childhood*, 21(1) 87–102.

Ochs, E. and Beck, M. (2013) Dinner. In E. Ochs and T. Kremer-Sadlik (eds.) *Fast Forward Family: Home Work and Relationships in Middle Class America.* Berkley: University of California Press.

Ochs, E. and Shohet, M. (2006) The cultural structuring of mealtime socialization. In Wiley Interscience (ed.) *New Direction for Child and Adolescent Development*, 111, Chapter 3, pp. 35–49.

Olsen, S. O. and Ruiz, S. (2008) Adolescents' influence in family meal decisions. *Appetite*, 51, 646–653.

Prout, A. (2005) *The Future of Childhood: Towards the Interdisciplinary Study of Children.* Oxon: Routledge, Falmer.

Qvortrup, J. (1987) Introduction. (Reprinted from The Sociology of Childhood). *International Journal of Sociology*, 17(3), 3–37.

Qvortrup, J. (2004) The waiting child, *Childhood: A Global Journal of Child Research*, 11(3), 267–273.

Romani, S. (2005) Feeding post-modern families: food preparation and consumption practices in new family structures. In K. M. Ekström and H. Brembeck (eds.) *European Advances in Consumer Research Volume 7.* Goteborg, Sweden: Association for Consumer Research, 250–254.

Sellerberg, A. (2008) En Het Potatis. Om mat och måltid i barn- och tonårsfamiljer, *Research reports in Sociology*, 3, Department of Sociology Lund University.

Short, F. (2003) Cooks, culinary ability and convenience food, *Petits Propos Culinaires*, 73, 45–54. Cited in Caraher 2004.

Sobal, J. and Nelson, M. K. (2003) Commensal eating patterns: a community study, *Appetite*, 41, 181–190.

Spiggle, S. (1994) Analysis and interpretation of qualitative data in consumer research, *Journal of Consumer Research*, 21(3), 491–503.

Valentine, G. (1999) Eating in home, consumption and identity, *The Sociological Review*, 47(3), 491–524.

van der Horst, K., Ferrage, A. and Rytz, A. (2014) Involving children in meal preparation. Effects on food intake, *Appetite*, 79(1), 18–24.

Ward, S. (1974) Consumer socialization, *Journal of Consumer Research*, 1(September), 1–16.

Warde, A. (1997) *Consumption, Food and Taste*. London: Sage.

Warde, A. (2016) *The Practice of Eating*. Cambridge: Polity Press.

Warren, E., Parry, O., Lynch, R. and Murphy, S. (2008) If I don't like it then I can choose what I want: Welsh school children's accounts of preference for and control over food choice, *Health Promotion International*, 23(2), 144–151.

Yates, L. and Warde, A. (2016) Eating together and eating alone: meal arrangements in British households, *British Journal of Sociology*, DOI: doi:10.1111/1468-4446.1223.

Zigler, E. and Child, I. L. (1969) Socialization. In G. Lindzey and E. Aronson (eds.) *The Handbook of Social Psychology*, 2nd edn., Vol. 2. *The Individual in a Social Context*. Reading, MA: Addison-Wesley. Cited in Wardet. al. 1974.

Part III

New Parenting Styles?

Chapter 9

When fathers feed their family
The emergence of new father roles in Denmark

Malene Gram and Alice Grønhøj

Introduction

These days, male consumers increasingly appear in printed and online media in new roles – pictured as engaged and caring fathers. Males displaying their status as involved fathers are particularly evident in social media: Dads increasingly appear with babies on Facebook (in Denmark at least), and are 'liked' by both men and women. An example of such a recent posting from a happy father read: 'The first week of paternity leave with this little nugget of gold has just flown past. Love [child's name],' accompanied by a picture of father with baby. This posting was followed by a host of comments such as '#dadonpaternityleave' and 'show us pictures of your other child, too', along with 71 likes. Another recent media entry stems from the British newspaper *The Guardian* where a journalist and new father has provided regular updates on his experiences with his firstborn son featuring under the name 'Man with a pram' (www.theguardian.com/lifeandstyle/series/man-with-a-pram), reflecting on the wonders of fatherhood and his son. These observations may indicate a significant shift in constructions of fathering allowing for more practical engagement with children, which also seems to entail a larger engagement with other tasks that were commonly delegated to the mother and wife previously, namely the 'mundane' household chores of grocery shopping, cooking and feeding the children.

Compared to what has been written about mothers and their feeding of children (DeVault, 1991; Bugge and Almås, 2006) and 'the positioning of mothers as "default parents"' (Nicholas Townsend's expression, 2002, quoted in Tanner et al., 2014, p. 209) for example in the literature on obesity issues among children, little has been written on fathers' engagement in the feeding of children (notable exceptions are Owen et al., 2010; Meah and Jackson, 2015). This is unsurprising as mothers are in general well-known to be more active in household chores everywhere, compared to fathers. However, this invisibility of fathers in relation to shopping for food, cooking and being concerned with the feeding of children is quite in contrast to what was found in a recent interview study in Denmark with 5–6-year-old children and their families. In a number of these families the fathers were very engaged or even in charge of shopping and cooking, and in doing and displaying family (Finch, 2007) in relation to food, thus not leaving these tasks to their partners. These findings give insights into relatively new father positions which have been more or less overlooked in the literature. Concern with the lack of interest in the father in family consumption is voiced in a number of recent studies (Owen et al., 2010; Tanner et al., 2014; Meah and Jackson, 2015; Schänzel and Smith, 2011; Schänzel and Jenkins, 2016). For scholars in academic fields such as the sociology of work (Gatrell & Cooper, 2008) and gender and family (Kaufman, 2013), the shifting gender roles have been discussed for some time.

Despite the fact that statistics show that in Denmark women also still tend to take on the majority of the housework, it is worthwhile taking a closer look at these emerging new and very active fathers as part of feeding and parenting practices in the family as this gives us a more thorough and full understanding of family life and eating practices in contemporary society.

This paper draws on the sparse research literature on father roles and fathers engaged in shopping, cooking and the feeding of their children. The Danish context of gender roles and work life patterns for mothers and fathers is sketched. Based on 11 family interviews, we explore how the father is presented and himself as often very active in mundane family chores. Finally, we reflect on the consequences of fathers being involved in these chores, and put forward the idea that this development may actually imply a reduction of possible father roles.

Literature review

To be a 'family' is a 'vitally important collective enterprise central to many consumption experiences' (Epp and Price, 2008, p. 50), and consumer socialization is thought to take place through social interaction between family members and can thus be observed through central everyday practices (Epp and Price, 2008). Furthermore, family food practices are important in the creation of healthy food habits in children (Holm, 2001; see Marshall, this volume). Still it is found that fathers have not been studied much when it comes to mundane everyday practices in the household.

In their article from 2014, through an analysis of the advertising in the magazine *Good Housekeeping* covering more than half a century, Marshall et al. report a move in depictions of fathers from one narrow father role in the 1950s as the breadwinner and provider, through a fragmentation of stable cultural scripts around fathering and masculinity, to a much broader array of possible father roles allowing for nurturing and caring, being emotionally engaged, responsible and accessible men through the later decades. In the advertisements from 2010, the most recent advertisements in their study, Marshall et al. find that fathers have become invisible, which the authors interpret as being caused by the recognition by advertisers that there are many possible forms of family, which makes a fixed father figure difficult to depict in advertisements. Therefore, the authors notice a focus on empowered female figures in relation to the family instead. They also find that even if fathers appear to be both more caring and more accessible, they are not depicted as particularly active in terms of household chores. Advertisements are arguably not a mirror of reality (Pollay, 1986), but still draw on possible and attractive cultural scripts, and they are therefore interesting to explore as representations of changes in society such as changes in gender roles, and — particularly relevant for this study – male positions in the home.

Few studies have been carried out focusing on the father's role in family shopping, cooking and feeding of children (exceptions are Owen et al., 2010; Meah and Jackson, 2015; Harrison et al., 2012). Some of these studies looked at fathers in families where fathers were single because of divorce or bereavement (Harrison et al., 2012), but very few studies have addressed two-parent families – and even fewer in wealthy contexts. Owen et al., 2010, included a group of affluent fathers in their study. They mainly addressed fathers by interviewing them alone, and found that fathers considered themselves involved in family food work, but a minority saw themselves as having the main responsibility or even doing their equal share. It was found that these fathers would strive to facilitate their children's food choices and agency through shopping and eating practices, also as a practical tactic to ensure that children get enough nourishment, which was considered to be more important than eating healthily. Fathers were well aware of dominant societal health discourses but a counter discourse was found in which they argued for their ability to ensure a healthy balance in their children's diet. The authors concluded that gendered patterns are shifting but still remain relatively stable.

Meah and Jackson (2015) studied fathers who were all fathers in blended families and all had experience with social parenting, where a non-biological parent is involved in some degree of parenting. Traditionally, fathers have been seen as providers of cash rather than of care (Featherstone, 2009 quoted in Meah and Jackson, 2015), and it has been suggested that 'men's contributions are organized in particularly masculine spaces of care – namely outside the domestic environment' (Meah and Jackson, 2015, p. 6 drawing on for example Barker, 2011). They found, however, that there is significant diversity in contemporary fathering practices, that lone fathering involves complex emotional geographies, and that their understandings of 'fathering' are linked both to their previous female partners and their own fathers (see Molander, this volume).

In an Australian study, Tanner et al. (2014) interviewed mothers about fathers. They found that:

assuming responsibility for the provision and preparation of family meals and caring for their children's health was mostly an unquestioned part of being a mother, and they found that the pressure of perceived judgment and expectations around the provision of healthy food, and effective management of children's weight, was palpable (p. 212).

The women in their study assumed 'primary, if not complete, responsibility for managing their family's diets, including attending to food preferences, shopping, planning and preparing family meals and feeding children' (p. 214). This was explained through practical circumstances such as fathers' absence due to work, poor cooking skills or dislike of cooking (p. 214). Furthermore, Tanner et al. (2014) found that 'Mothers often emphasized partners' willingness to help whilst stressing their own superior expertise and enjoyment of cooking (p. 214), and being 'more expert and more "healthy" than fathers' (p 215), whereas fathers were perceived by the mothers to be peripheral to feeding the family.

Methodology

The present paper is based on an interview study from 2013, where we interviewed 35 5–6-year-olds in five kindergartens in relatively wealthy areas around two Danish cities to find out more about children's participation in family decisions on healthy and unhealthy food (Gram and Grønhøj, 2015; Gram and Grønhøj, 2016). A letter of consent was distributed to parents through the kindergarten leaders, and in this letter families were asked to sign up for family interviews to supplement interviews with the children. 14 families volunteered, and 13 families (one email address did not work) were interviewed afterwards, including the children, who were thus interviewed twice (except one child who was ill on the day of the kindergarten visit). Fathers participated in 11 family interviews (in one family the parents were divorced and in another family the father was away on a business trip). We were surprised to see the level of engagement and participation among most of the fathers who took part in the interviews. As described in the introductory part, this level of involvement and participation is under-described in the literature, and we therefore decided to explore this perspective further. The present article therefore draws on the family interviews only, and only when the fathers took part. To ensure the anonymity of the participants, pseudonyms are used. The fathers in the study spanned from 33 to 54 years in age and almost all had long tertiary educations. They represented an almost equal amount of fathers of boys and girls, and the majority had more than one child (see Table 9.1).

All interviews were carried out by the two authors. The first interview was carried out with both authors to discuss and adjust the interview guide and the interview techniques (small exercises, use of a video clip, and vignettes to

Table 9.1 Overview of sample and assessment of participation

Father	Shopping	Cooking	Part. in Socialisation	Age	Employment
Anders	(X)	?	X	45	folk high school teacher
Flemming	X	X	X	37	logistics and energy
Esben	X	X	X	38	engineer
Mikkel	**X**	**X**	X	34	just finished master degree
Lars	**X**	X	X	43	sales representative
Jacob	X	X	X	42	engineer
Jørgen	(X)	?	(X)	54	head of highschool
Kim	X	(X)	X	43	project manager
Peter	X	X	X	33	football agent
Christian	X	?	X	36	project manager
Poul	X	X	X	44	system developer

Notes: x = participation, (x) = some participation, **x** = major responsibility, ? = not known

stimulate talk). The subsequent interviews were carried out by one author at a time, followed by a discussion of field notes and preliminary analysis with the absent author. Interviews with families were carried out in their homes, at their kitchen/dining tables, in most cases with all family members participating. Interviews lasted between 40 and 70 minutes, and addressed issues such as family food shopping, healthy/unhealthy food choices, and parent-child negotiations. The father's role in the family was not addressed specifically but appeared from the family interviews and through their own and their partners' descriptions of their participation in everyday practices.

Data was analyzed through thematic analysis as described by Kvale (1996). The sparse literature on fathers' engagement in family food practices and shopping was explored at the same time as interviews were carried out, and the data was scrutinized through an iterative hermeneutic process to understand the fathers' role in the family in relation to food shopping, cooking and engagement in the children's food socialization.

Tanner et al. (2014) chose to study fathers' roles through interviews with mothers. In the present study it is a clear advantage that fathers' voices are included directly. It is a limitation, however, that we did not address the issue of the position of the father directly, and that we did not ask fathers to reflect on their role in household chores. It strengthens the argument of a more visible father role, however, that fathers' participation in household chores still became very visible through the interviews.

Furthermore, that fact that families were interviewed together is considered an important strength. Being interviewed with a non-member of the family present, a clear 'frontstage' situation (Goffman, 1959) is created where impressions are managed and the family is displayed (Finch, 2007). This could have meant that partners were not eager to be open about their own and each other's efforts in the household. The fact, though, that the interviews included the whole family together at a time, meant that particularly children would address statements which were not in tune with how they perceived family reality which is similar to the advantage of interviewing friendship groups in focus groups. Thus, close acquaintances are likely to perform social control when met with information they cannot recognize from their usual day-to-day interaction (Halkier, 2003). For this reason we argue that it would not have been possible for a father to pretend that he often goes to the supermarket with the child if this was not the case. The power hierarchy among children and adults in Denmark, particularly in well-educated families, is usually low and anti-authoritarian, and we find it unlikely that children would not speak their minds. Moreover, the fathers' participation in housework was often narrated through concrete examples of, for example, the child and father shopping or cooking together. The family interview setting, including the children, thus seems to have ensured a clear connection between talk and reflections of participation and actual 'real' participation and thus appears to have validated the statements of the interviewees. Still a certain level of 'sugar-coating' may have taken place when the family is displaying itself. Furthermore, because house work is mundane and routinized, it risks being so much part of habit that it may be difficult to account for. Still, accounts of everyday situations (e.g. 'Tell me about the last time you went to the supermarket with your child') gave good insights into the fathers' participation and positions. Furthermore, techniques specifically aimed at retrieving so-called low involvement, everyday practices, such as vignettes, that is, short stories of common, everyday situations, for instance when shopping in the supermarket, were also applied (Grønhøj & Bech-Larsen, 2010).

This present study focused on fathering practices in families where both parents are living in the households, and, in contrast to several previous studies, not in times of conflict, disruption, or lack of financial means. The study includes voices of both fathers and mothers.

Danish parents have good conditions to reconcile work and family. There is an extensive system of public care for children, and in a European setting a relatively long maternity leave is offered along with good possibilities for paternity leave even though few fathers use this option (http://eige.europa.eu/ sites/default/files/documents/a_hug_from_daddy_denmark_awareness-raising. pdf). Household tasks are gender biased in Denmark as in all of Europe, but according to a recent EU report tasks are perceived as more equally shared than in other European countries. The amount of hours spent on household chores does not differ much across Europe among women, but the number of hours put in by men do differ. While women in all countries find that they do more than their fair share, men admit that they do less than their fair share (p. 10). When replying to the question 'Do you think the share of the household work you do is just about fair', 80% of Danish women answer yes, compared to 58% of UK women and 22% of French women, in 2010 (http://www.eurofound.europa.eu/pubdocs/2010/02/en/1/EF1002EN. pdf). In Denmark the number of working hours outside the home per week is among the lowest in Europe and the highest percentage do telework from home which is seen as easing the work–life balance.

Findings

Among the 11 fathers interviewed in this study, most of them were engaged in shopping, cooking and their children's feeding. Most fathers were participating significantly, and some were even found to be in charge of both grocery shopping and cooking in their family. To get an overview of the estimated level of involvement assessed through the family interviews, see Table 9.1. The issue and level of fathers' participation was not addressed directly in the interviews, and for this reason we were not able to assess the level of participation of all participants, but for most fathers their level of participation became clear through their accounts. Above, fathers' participation in household tasks is marked with an 'x'. If their participation was very high it is marked with a bold 'x', if their participation was minor it is marked with (x). If it did not become clear during the interview whether or not the fathers participated it is marked with a question mark.

The parents in the interviews most often seemed to agree on their policies on food and on their descriptions of how their everyday lives in relation to food and children play out, even though in a few families some tension and mild reproaching of the other could be observed. While a couple of men remained relatively passive during the interviews, letting their partners take the lead, the majority of fathers were very active during the interviews. They were eager to explain how they include children in supermarket visits, what is important for them when they shop and cook, and the ideas they have developed to avoid conflict in the supermarket when shopping with children and to ensure that their children eat a varied diet. Through their accounts they often demonstrated how doing household chores are an immanent part of their practices. An example of this stems from the interview with Lars' family. Lars, the father, does most of the shopping, most often with his son Rasmus, who is 5:

> Well, he is a very independent guy, too, so if I ask him to find hay for the guinea pigs, then he will bring back hay for the guinea pigs. And he remembers, too, if I have said in the morning, we need tin foil wrapping for the packed lunches. Then he has just picked that up on the way.

The quote illustrates not just that going shopping with his son is a frequently occurring practice but also that the father is engaged in preparing packed lunches in the morning and planning ahead what to buy. He also shows that he is impressed with his son, and that he notices his independence. As with the example from Lars above, through their accounts fathers illustrate that they are involved in the nitty-gritty everyday issues related to the feeding of their children. Another example of this is Esben's explanation of how they deal with children who are very hungry when they get home from kindergarten and then not hungry at dinnertime:

> When they come home from kindergarten, then they call for food, and then sometimes an apple or something is cut up for them. But then we also know that there we have some kind of a dilemma. We would rather not feed them, because then they're not hungry when we sit at dinner, which we'll really like them to, also eating and not just sitting there. But if they are super hungry, and are just about dying and nag, and are really irritating because they nag for blueberries or apples or bananas, or something, luckily mostly fruit. Then they sometimes get that. We know this costs on the appetite half an hour or three quarters of an hour later. If it's then not there [the appetite], then we end up concluding that it's going to be all right, that they have eaten an apple.

This quote illustrates also that Esben is fully familiar with and addresses the healthy eating discourse by his insertion 'luckily mostly fruit' in opposition to biscuits, sweets or similar. He is deeply engaged in the practical dilemma of having either a hungry and hard-to-deal-with child or a content child who is then not hungry for his or her dinner. Furthermore, he simultaneously addresses the issue that most parents stress as a very important socialization goal for their children and part of the family enterprise: sitting together at the end of the day and sharing a meal together and 'not just sitting there'.

While all fathers in the study engage in food shopping, some of the fathers are the main purchasers in the family. Mikkel, for instance, takes full responsibility for shopping and cooks almost all family meals.

WIFE: You're best at grocery shopping, Mikkel. We have to say that.
M: We can easily say that.
INTERVIEWER: Why is he the best at that?
M: [to wife]: You never know what we have, you just shop.
WIFE: It's Mikkel, who almost always cooks and clearly has the best overview of what's in the kitchen.

While Mikkel describes his wife as lacking in food shopping skills and lacking overview what is needed at home – to which she fully agrees – he takes on the main responsibility of both shopping and cooking. Furthermore, he often brings his young daughters to the supermarket.

Several fathers exemplify how they have learnt how to avoid conflicts with their children in supermarkets by involving their children in fetching goods, by letting them carry goods and by avoiding going to the supermarket when both children and they themselves are tired. These practices illustrate that fathers' engagement is ongoing. They have had experiences and they have adjusted their practices which according to themselves are relatively unproblematic. Furthermore, several fathers seem very aware of what their children like to eat, and several are willing to forgo food items they only like themselves (strong cheese, Lars; steaks, Esben) to avoid food waste or that other family members will not eat an evening meal with these ingredients. While concerned with healthy eating, several fathers seem particularly engaged in food socialization with regards to the importance of having a holistic view on eating (cf. Gram and Grønhøj, 2015), underlining the importance of enjoying food, and not to become fanatically health-oriented.

Also during the interviews several fathers demonstrated that they were used to engaging closely with their children. For instance, Emil is losing his patience during the interview, and his father says 'Emil, will you come over and sit with daddy?' in an attempt to distract him and calm him down, in this way taking responsibility for the boy's behaviour in the interview situation and acting on it.

While most fathers' involvement with shopping, cooking and their children's food socialization was noticeable and substantial, a few fathers appeared to assume a more detached role. An example of this was the interview with Jørgen whose wife was clearly taking the lead in these feeding activities, at the same time as she was much more frequently approached by the children during the interview with regard to various food requests and comments about the family's daily food related activities.

Summing up, several fathers in this study were clearly very engaged in household chores and caring for their children at the practical as well as emotional levels, a finding which was substantiated by observations in the interviews: we heard 'accounts of action' (Halkier, 2003) when fathers explained about their involvement in feeding their children and observed 'accounts in action' (Halkier, 2003) when fathers were actively attending to their children during the interviews. Most fathers demonstrated significant knowledge of what children preferred and what it would take to ensure that they eat healthily. Several fathers were in charge of shopping, often engaging their young children in finding goods, just as several fathers were in charge of cooking and very engaged in food quality, healthy eating and a few also with environmental concerns such as carbon footprint. Several demonstrated through their narratives that they think and plan ahead in relation to meals to come, even though managing the household at this level has often been ascribed to mothers (DeVault, 1991).

Discussion and conclusion

The aim of this chapter was to explore father roles in relation to shopping, cooking and feeding of children in the family. In contrast to the literature that mainly addresses mothers as interviewees and as the main responsible person when it comes to food in families with children (for example Bugge and Almås, 2006; DeVault, 1991), this study shows that fathers are not just distant figures, standing on the sideline or even being counterproductive to their children's healthy eating as they are to some extent depicted for example by Tanner et al., 2014. The fathers in this study take on very active roles and responsibility in relation to chores often ascribed to women. It seems to be an advantage that this study is based on interviews where fathers, mothers and children participated as this becomes a discussion of joint practices. Unlike Owen et al.'s 2010 study we find that among our group of men it was the majority who did take part in household chores, even though fathers co-habited with the child/ren/'s mother, and as part of what appears to be a genuine sharing of tasks rather than because the mother was unable to do it herself. This may be linked to the Scandinavian context, to the relatively high social class in focus in this study and a move towards less of a contradiction between masculinity and partaking in housework chores.

Epp and Price (2008) emphasize the importance of everyday interaction of family members in the ongoing creation of family identity. This study shows that several of the fathers are very active in their participation and engagement with their children through mundane household practices in a way which has not been exposed much in earlier writings on fathers and household chores.

In Marshall et al.'s (2014) study, the most recent years of analysis of the father role seen through ads showed an invisible father. A fixed father role in this period of time was found to be difficult to depict by advertisers. Marshall et al. found that from a narrow depiction of the father as a distant breadwinner and provider in the 1950s, there is an opening for a much broader array of positions for fathers in the ads also including caring roles and fathers being accessible. At no time in the ads, however, Marshall et al.

found male figures particularly involved in mundane housework. Recent movements in society demonstrate a larger involvement of fathers in caring for family and children, also on a more practical and mundane basis, and these movements are perhaps particularly outspoken in the Danish context, as reflected in the media and statistics on gender roles, and also recognized in the present study. One could even argue that the very broad range of possible father positions sketched by Marshall et al. is being reduced again, as the distant breadwinner father is no longer a figure which seems relevant or possible, particularly in the Danish context, where most women are also breadwinners. In the same vein, *not* participating in practical household chores such as shopping, cooking and caring for children does not seem to be an option either. The fathers interviewed in this study appear to find this participation both 'natural' and for several even enjoyable and something they are passionate about.

No doubt the sharing of mundane household chores is still unequal, as found by Owen et al. (2010), but if fathering practices are only or mainly reported through mothers (as suggested by Aitken, 2005 quoted in Meah and Jackson, 2015), there may be a risk that – just as women's housework has been seen as invisible and therefore often undervalued (DeVault, 1991) – men's housework may risk being invisible, too. Certainly, if their voices are not heard in research, fathers' contributions will remain under-explored. The present study attests that several of the fathers interviewed indeed take on responsibility in cooperation with their partners to make family life flow, because they want to play a role in their children's lives with the aim of helping their children develop robust eating habits and, more generally, to see them grow up to be healthy, independent persons. Still this does by no means signify that inequality is gone. Societal norms still render mothers' participation usual, normal and expected as for example reported by Tanner et al. (2014), while fathers doing the same is less usual and not expected in the same way – and perhaps fathers' participation receives more credit for less work. Finally, active fathering is possibly followed with less stress and guilt than mothering (Davies et al., 2010), which is something which would be interesting to explore in further depth.

The Danish context of this study probably means that the division of household tasks is more equally shared and thus perhaps more progressive than in many other countries. The findings are somewhat at odds with what is found in literature based on non-Scandinavian data (for example Tanner et al., 2014). We interpret this as being closely linked to the Scandinavian context in which an early gender liberation movement directed the public's attention to the significance of (women's) unpaid work at home, and which also had a strong focus on the importance of granting paternity leave. This may be seen as precursor of the now longstanding societal concern of including the father in childcare which is reflected in this study's active participation by fathers.

We argue that it is important to recognize this more active role of fathers in Denmark as part of everyday practices in relation to for example societal objectives of creating changes in family diets to encourage healthier eating.

References

Aitken, S. (2005). Fathering and faltering: 'Sorry, but you don't have the necessary accoutrements'. *Environment and Planning A*, 32, 581–598.

Barker, J. (2011). 'Manic mums' and 'distant dads'? Gendered geographies of care and the journey to school. *Health and Place*, 17, 413–421.

Bugge, A.B. & Almås, R. (2006). Domestic dinner: Representations and practices of a proper meal among young suburban mothers. *Journal of Consumer Culture*, 6, 203.

Davies, A., Dobscha, S., Geiger, S., O'Donohue, S., O'Malley, L., Prothero, A. & Sorensen, E.B. (2010). Buying into motherhood? Problematic consumption and ambivalence in transitional phases. *Consumption, Markets and Culture*. 13(4), 373–397.

DeVault, M. (1991). *Feeding the Family: The Social Organization of Caring as Gendered Work*. Chicago: Chicago University Press.

Epp, A.M. & Price, L.L. (2008). Family identity. A framework of identity interplay in consumption practices. *Journal of Consumer Research*. 35, 50–70.

Featherstone, B. (2009). *Contemporary Fathering: Theory, Policy and Practice*. Cambridge: Polity.

Finch, J. (2007) Displaying families. *Sociology*, 41(1), 65–81.

Gatrell, C.J. & Cooper, C.L. (2008). Work-life balance: Working for whom? *European Journal of International Management*, 2(1), 71–86.

Goffman, E. (1959). *The Presentation of Self in Everyday Life*. New York: Doubleday.

Gram, M. & Grønhøj, A. (2015). 'There is usually just one Friday a week': Parents and children's categorizations of 'unhealthy' food. *Food, Culture and Society*. 18(4), 547–567.

Gram, M. & Grønhøj, A. (2016). 'Meet the good child'. 'Childing' practices in family food shopping. *International Journal of Consumer Studies*. doi:10.1111/ijcs.12295.

Grønhøj, A. & Bech-Larsen, T. (2010). Using vignettes to study family consumption processes. *Psychology & Marketing*, 27(5), 445–464.

Halkier, B. (2003). *Fokusgrupper*. Samfundslitteratur: København.

Harrison, R., Gentry, J. W. & Commuri, S. (2012). A Grounded Theory of Transition to Involved Parenting: The Role of Household Production and Consumption in the Lives of Single Fathers. In Cele Otnes and Linda Tuncay Zayer (ed.), *Gender, Culture, and Consumer Behavior*(pp. 337–370). London: Routledge.

Holm, L. (2001). Family meals. In U. Kjærnes (ed.): *Eating Patterns: A Day in the Lives of Nordic People* (pp. 199–212). Norway: Nation Institute for Consumer Research.

Kaufman, G. (2013). *Superdads: How Fathers Balance Work and Family in the 21st Century*. New York: NYU Press.

Kvale, S. (1996). *Interviews*. London: SAGE Publications.

Marshall, D., Davis, T., Hogg, M. K., Schneider, T. & Petersen, A. (2014). From overt provider to invisible presence: Discursive shifts in advertising portrayals of the father in Good Housekeeping, 1950–2010. *Journal of Marketing Management*, 30 (15–16), 1654–1679.

Meah, A. & Jackson, P. (2015). The complex landscape of contemporary fathering in the UK. *Social & Cultural Geography*. doi:10.1080/14649365.2015.1089586.

Owen, J., Metcalfe, A. et al. (2010). 'If they don't eat it, it's not a proper meal': Images of risk and choice in fathers' accounts of family food practices. *Health, Risk & Society*, 12(4), 395–406.

Pollay, R.W. (1986). The distorted mirror: reflections on the unintended consequences of advertising. *Journal of Marketing*, 50(2), 18–36.

Schänzel, H. & Jenkins, J. (2016). Non-resident fathers' holidays alone with their children: Experiences, meanings and fatherhood. *World Leisure Journal*, doi:10.1080/16078055.2016.1216887.

Schänzel, H. & Smith, K.A. (2011). The absence of fatherhood: Achieving true gender scholarship in family tourism research. *Annals of Leisure Research*. 14(2–3), 143–154.

Tanner, C., Petersen, A. & Fraser, S. (2014). Food, fat and family: Thinking fathers through mothers' words. *Women's Studies International Forum* 44, 2009–2219.

Townsend, N. (2002) *The Package Deal: Marriage, Work and Fatherhood in Men's Lives*. Philadelphia: Temple University Press.

Chapter 10

Swedish single fathers feeding the family

Susanna Molander

Introduction

Cooking plays a pivotal role in everyday life, particularly in relation to caring for children (cf. DeVault 1991; Lupton 1996; Molander 2011). The aim of this chapter is to elucidate cooking among Swedish single fathers—a group that has increased their engagement with their children substantially during the last 30 years (SCB 2014). However, with some interesting exceptions of studies based in a North American context (e.g. Coskuner-Balli and Thompson 2013; Harrison, Gentry and Commuri 2012) we still know relatively little about men's childcare and associated consumption on an everyday basis—a practice that presumably will have a strong impact on society in the future and where some of the forerunners can be found among single fathers. These often, well-educated, middle-class fathers, usually working full-time while also being responsible for child rearing and household chores, embody 'dual emancipation'—a long held ideal in the Swedish gender equality debate. Dual emancipation implies that both men and women should have equal access to work life and care work and thereby be emancipated from their pre-described gender roles (Klinth 2002), which makes them relevant to study as the vanguard for a new era of fathers.

Although Sweden is seen as a relatively gender equal country by most commentators, women still take main responsibility for most of the care of the children, the household and the associated consumption (Duvander, Ferrarini and Johansson 2015; Forsberg 2009; Plantin 2015; SCB 2010). But even if caregiving fathers have become more common in Sweden, expectations of them are lower and skepticism of their care is higher than for mothers (cf. Mellström 2006; Östberg 2012; Plantin 2003).

In light of the growing number of caregiving fathers, the following study explores sixteen Swedish single fathers cooking for their children. The chapter begins with a theoretical overview of fatherhood in a state of flux. It continues with findings that first point to some general results and then elaborate on the fathers' different approaches to cooking. It ends with a concluding discussion pointing to a relatively laidback and pragmatic approach to cooking—an approach that also characterized their relationship with the market.

Fatherhood in a state of flux

Even after 40 years of state intervention regarding gender equality in work and family, including generous parental leave, the Nordic countries still have a long way to go before they have achieved their goals. Though a caring father is certainly an ideal in the Nordic context (Brandth and Kvande 2013), this ideal has still not had the practical impact envisioned by politicians (Duvander, Ferrarini and Johansson 2015; Plantin 2015). Nordic men admittedly spend more time at home than before, but they generally remain the main provider, while women work part-time and still take primary responsibility for childcare and household chores (Duvander, Ferrarini and Johansson 2015; Forsberg 2009; Plantin 2003). One reason for this slow development despite generous Nordic parental leave is said to be the continued stereotyped expectations of what is male or female (Mellström 2006) and that working life is still central to the way masculinity is constructed (ibid.). In this competitive "marketplace masculinity" (Kimmel 2013, 228) men are often depicted as men of action, handling the world in a rational and efficient way (Holt and Thompson 2004; Ross-Smith and Kornberger 2004).

Changes can, however, be discerned among the Nordic young educated middle class who increasingly choose to stay at home during part of their children's first year (Duvander, Ferrarini and Johansson 2015; Försäkringskassan 2013) and who in the case of divorce increasingly share responsibility for the child's residence, upbringing and care (SCB 2014). Research suggests that the earmarked parental leave quotas have influenced the increase in fathers taking the opportunity to experience the daily wear and tear of parenthood and what it really means to be an involved parent (Brandth and Kvande 2013). The enhanced status of the child (Beck and Beck-Gernsheim 1995; Miller 1998) and masculinity's rising emotionalization (Mellström 2006) point to a continuation of this development.

Studies on consuming fathers from an Anglo-Saxon context, however, describe more traditional fatherhood practices. Here, stay-at-home fathers seek to enhance the cultural legitimacy for their marginalized gender identity through various types of manly consumption (Coskuner-Balli and Thompson 2013). Research suggests that divorced fathers lack support from consumer society during the tough transition to single fatherhood (Harrison, Gentry and Commuri 2012); and that although they engage in more childcare, representations of the father as breadwinner and protector continues to dominate popular culture and advertising (Gentry and Harrison 2010; Marshall, Davis, Hogg, Schneider, and Petersen 2015; Robinson and Hunter 2008). While very informative, the Anglo-Saxon political and cultural context differs greatly from that of the fathers in this study. The Swedish fathers studied here live in a context that is generally more endorsing of fathers' engagement in everyday childcare and which supports men seeking to combine full time work with child rearing. When exploring the different routes that fatherhood may take in the future, Swedish single middle-class fathers are especially interesting to study firstly considering that Sweden has a positive image internationally as far as gender equality is concerned (World Economic Forum 2014), and secondly considering that these single working and caring fathers can be seen as the vanguard of the long held Swedish ideal of dual emancipation.

Culinary femininities and masculinities

Cooking and all the other activities surrounding feeding the family, including planning, purchasing, preparing and cleaning up, are usually seen as part of women's devotional duty and caring work; and a way to reinforce the family identity and her position within it (DeVault 1991; Lupton 1996; Miller 1998; Moisio et al. 2004; Molander 2011; Wilk 2010). This care includes sacrifices such as self-abnegating one's own desires while prioritizing others' preferences and requests (Cappellini and Parsons 2012). The need for sacrifice is also highlighted through the tension between care and convenience as it emerges as less caring to buy ready-made food than by intermingling it with labor—convenience is simply the antithesis to 'homely love' (Warde 1997, 132–133). While some argue that the emergent ideology of intensive mothering entailing a wholly child-centered, emotionally involving practice might increase the demands for self-sacrifice even further (Hays 1996), others contend that mothers are also pragmatic and able to negotiate between ideals and what is practically possible (Carrigan and Szmigin 2006; Gram and Pedersen 2014; Cairns et al. this volume).

However, today cooking has also become an increasingly accepted part of what fathers do, both in the Nordic countries (Aarseth and Olsen 2008; Ekström 2016; Neuman, Gottzén and Fjellström 2015) and elsewhere (Szabo 2013, 2014). Men are usually said to have the choice and flexibility in relation to housework and care (Bekkenger 2003) and their cooking is typically perceived as leisure or play (Klasson and Ulver 2015). While women generally have primary responsibility for everyday cooking, men cook on special occasions (Szabo 2013). According to Szabo (2014), in the literature "traditional culinary masculinities" have generally been described as oriented towards cooking as a practical skill, as culinary art/performance, as leisure, and as a strategy for (heterosexual) seduction. This is opposed to the "traditional culinary femininities" approach to cooking that is said to be more focused on love and care. "Traditional culinary masculinities" are furthermore described as having an easy-going, low-anxiety approach to nutrition, while women experience more anxiety. Rather than dichotomizing men's and women's cooking even further, Szabo (2014), however, finds that the more experience men have in feeding others, the more they orient towards love, care and anxiety (see Gram and Grønhøj, this volume). Also Neuman, Gottzén and Fjellström (2015) argue for a reconsideration of the dichotomization. Their study on Swedish men's cooking highlights that whether cooking is fun or not, it has become a self-evident part of men's life and that a desirable gender equal masculinity is one with cooking skills beyond survival level.

Overall, there has been a growing interest in cooking in Sweden. Today, food is not only about survival and care, but increasingly about health, beauty, trend, refinement, style and, well, anything that can be captured in the word 'status.' In fact, thanks to the last 30 years of Swedish gastronomic revolution (Jönsson 2012)—including a greater interest in sophisticated cooking and dining out—domestic cooking has been gaining legitimacy among Swedish men without any accompanying emasculation (Neuman, Gottzén and Fjellström 2015). Indeed, this low status domestic work that for centuries has been practiced by women is now inspired by, and gains status from, a gastronomy that for centuries has been dominated by men (Neuman and Fjellström 2014). But while we know that more and more men are cooking for reasons of pleasure, increased status and increased gender equality (Neuman, Gottzén and Fjellström 2015), there is still a need to know more about how it is performed in relation to masculinities in everyday settings (Klasson och Ulver 2015), particularly among men belonging to the vanguard of dual emancipation with access to both work life and care.

Method

The chapter focuses on the food and cooking aspects discussed in a larger study based on interviews and diaries concerning the everyday lives of a group of sixteen single middle-class fathers, with social class here referring to a certain grade of education and occupation. The data on food and cooking could therefore also relate to the men's life-worlds as a whole. Based on existential phenomenology, primacy was placed on the perspective of the fathers and how their life-worlds and experiences were interrelated (Thompson, Locander and Pollio 1989). The fathers were recruited through an organization for single parents and a request on social media. After an initial interview which provided an introduction to the fathers and their lives, they carried out a diary study for 7 days. Similar to Facebook updates, they were asked to describe their lives as fathers through the various activities they carried out with help of two photographs a day along with a short description of the type of activity each photograph referred to as well as their thoughts about the activity. The diaries were then followed up through autodriving (Heisley and Levy 1991) where the fathers were encouraged to comment on and discuss the situations represented in the diaries and were also asked complementary questions.

The data set consists of photographs and texts describing the various activities they performed as fathers along with transcribed interviews. Using an existential phenomenological approach (Thompson, Locander and Pollio 1989), and with their general profiles as a backdrop, data covering everything related to food and cooking was analyzed in an iterative process guided by the research objective to elucidate the fathers cooking for their children in relation to their lives as a whole. The reading of relevant theoretical material guided initial readings of the data, and was followed by subsequent data analysis, interpretation, and rereading of the literature. A description of the sixteen fathers who participated in the study can be found in Table 10.1.

Findings

Still breadwinners

The fathers in this study were, with a few exceptions, firmly anchored in their professional identities. Engaged in areas such as IT, engineering, finance, advertising, management consulting and public office, none of them seemed to have given up advancing their careers. Even if most of them said that they had put their careers somewhat on hold now that their childrearing was so intense, only one of them spoke about scaling down, selling the house and working as a sailing instructor once his kids had grown older. Some had shared custody and they had extra help from public childcare, a temporary babysitter or sometimes grandparents. Like Hochschild's (1989) 'second shift'—referring to the housework, childcare and household management tasks that women usually deal with before and after their paid work—this was to a large part what the fathers were also engaged in when not working.

However, these working fathers did not seem stigmatized by domestic work in the same way as the caring stay-at-home fathers in Coskuner-Balli and Thompson's (2013) study. Those fathers tried to break free from both breadwinner masculinity and the feminizing connotations historically associated with domesticity through masculinizing practices—which meant re-situating their domestic responsibilities in the public sphere, putting more emphasis on the technological aspects of domestic work as well as to a higher degree outsourcing responsibility for meal preparation to the commercial marketplace. Although some of these masculinizing practices could be attributed to the fathers in this study as well, domestic work did not emerge as threatening. This was probably because one of the major building blocks of the masculine identities of the men in this study remained intact, namely that of the breadwinner.

Table 10.1 Participants' profile

Name	Age	Work	Children*	Custody	Diary
Erik	40s	IT consultant	1 girl & 1 boy (grade)	Sole	7 days
Thomas	40s	IT consultant	3 girls (2 grade, 1 teen)	Sole	7 days
Dante	40s	Financial advisor	1 girl (grade)	Sole	7 days
Mikael	40s	Engineer	1girl & 1 boy (pre)	Sole	7 days
Per	40s	Public official	2 boys (pre, teen)	Joint**	6 days
Johan	30s	Project manager	1 girl (pre)	Joint	5 days
Magnus	40s	NGO consultant	1 girl (grade)	Joint	7 days
Jonas	40s	Student/ Businessman	1 girl (teen), 1 boy (grade)	Joint	5 days
Anders	40s	NGO official	1 girl (teen)	Joint	7 days
Karl	30s	Financial advisor	1 boy (toddler)	Joint	7 days
Björn	50s	IT consultant	2 boys (grade, young adult)	Joint	4 days
Klas	50s	Management consultant	4 boys (2 grade, 1 teen, 1 y adult)	Joint	7 days
Hans	50s	Consultant	2 girls (teen, grade), 1 boy (teen)	Joint	7 days
Ulf	40s	Advertising consultant	1 girl (teen), 1 boy (grade)	Joint	6 days
Daniel	30s	Healthcare worker	1 girl (grade), 2 boys (grade, teen)	Joint	5 days
Bo	50s	Management consultant	2 girls (teen), 2 boys (pre, teen)	Joint	7 days

** Per had joint custody, but in practice sole as his partner was very sick.

The fathers' cooking was part of a never-ending flow of activities including working, dropping off, picking up and taking part in their children's various activities, shopping, engaging in various household chores, helping children with their homework and putting them to bed. Since their work took so much of their time, they had to organize their lives as efficiently as possible and most of them seemed assured that they did the best they could. On the whole, while striving for efficiency, most of the men emerged as functionally oriented and pragmatic and they did not seem to ponder very much about food.

Cooking is a major part of being a father

Although approached in different ways, cooking was an essential part of the men's parenting. Most of them usually had dinner with their children and more than half also emphasized that they involved their children in the cooking. The study included photos showing small hands cutting green beans and running mini-shopping trolleys along with stories about children helping out with making meatballs, pancakes or being in charge of the food once a week. This involvement is also in line with other research that points out that children's role to some extent changes after a divorce, and that the children then help out to a greater extent (Bates and Gentry1994; Molander 2011; Tinson, Nancarrow and Brace 2008).

The fact that cooking has reached new heights (Jönsson 2012) was also evident in this study. As many as eight of the sixteen fathers more or less explicitly described their interest in cooking and health and this is the group I call 'Cooking as an interest.' Only four of the fathers emerged as more traditional father figures portraying 'Cooking as a hardship.' The remaining four fathers did not seem to consider cooking a nuisance or a great interest, and this is the group I call 'Cooking as a part of life.' Each of these groups will be further elaborated on below.

Cooking as an interest

> Well, for me food is important; how it's produced, that I buy and cook food that contains all the necessary nutrients. I'm interested in exercise and diet and eat a lot of food that I think is supposed to be wholesome. And this is also something I try to reflect in what she [my daughter] eats, even though I am much stricter with myself than with her. So I guess I have some kind of philosophy that says it's much better if children eat food than sweets.
>
> (Johan, interview)

Over the last years, there has been an increased interest in the body, food and health (Spicer and Cederström 2015) and this is also apparent in the data. Among the eight fathers who expressed an explicit interest in food and cooking, five also connected it to their interest in health and sports as reflected in Johan's quote above. There are several aspects that make this quote interesting as a comparison to what is usually considered to be "traditional culinary femininities" (Szabo 2014).

Firstly, rather than considering cooking a sacrifice, self-abnegating one's own desires and prioritizing others' preferences and requests (Cappellini and Parsons 2012), Johan's approach to food and cooking was based on his own interest in exercise and diet. The own autonomous self emerged as more distinct than in studies on women whose identity to a higher degree is linked to their children and being a mother (Hays 1996; Molander 2011; Rich 1986). Even if Johan said he tried to reflect his view of food in his daughter's eating it did not seem like a big deal if this was not successful in practice. Though trying to make her buy into his way of eating, Johan and his daughter came out as two different individuals. This autonomy was in fact something that most of the fathers with an interest in food and cooking expressed. Although they in varying degrees wanted their children to eat as they did, it was not their role as parents that seemed to have ignited this concern, but rather a general interest in health or food and cooking in itself.

Secondly, and like most fathers in this study, although Johan was set on having dinner with his child every evening during their weeks together, his focus on nutrients made his approach to food appear more functionally oriented than is generally seen when mothers are involved (Bugge and Almås 2006; Cappellini and Parsons 2012; DeVault 1991; Miller 1998; Moisio, Arnould and Price 2004; Molander 2011). This approach was also shared by Björn, whose youngest son (grade-schooler) did a lot of sports. Björn was always concerned about making sure his son got the proper nourishment before running off to his various activities and had cut out sugar by changing ice cream for yoghurt and candies for nuts and fruits. But even when they showed an interest in the aesthetics and pleasures related to cooking and eating, such fathers seemed to be more concerned about proper nourishment. For example, Karl began cooking as a teenager, ran a restaurant after finishing his university studies and was now the owner of a restaurant alongside his position as a financial advisor:

> Every good meal has three components [carbohydrates, proteins and vegetables] / ... / and then, considering the various possibilities you have to combine these [components], you can basically construct an abundance of dishes while still having a good mix [of them] and offer fruit afterwards.

In general, rather than talking about food in terms of aesthetics and pleasure they discussed it in terms of nutrients. Erik was an exception by emphasizing how much he enjoyed grilling meat and preparing home grown potatoes after work in the sun in his own backyard: "That's quality of life for me!"

While vegetables used to be linked to femininity (Lupton 1996, 109), they have increasingly been associated with health and therefore seen as something that men can also relate to. Health has become a status object that together with a well-toned body is said to be an increasingly important means of competition in society (Cederström and Spicer 2015). Virtually all fathers urged their children to eat vegetables and broccoli was a favorite among quite a few of the children. As opposed to Lupton who discussed "food as fuel" only in relation to people with very little interest in food (1996, 143–144), in this study food emerged as fuel also among the fathers interested in cooking. It seemed to be a way to refuel the engine before running off to the next thing and was only one part of their overall care for their children—care that usually included far more than food and which was often related to sports, the ultimate embodiment of masculinity (Kimmel 2012). There were, however, exceptions of fathers who rather than nourishment explicitly emphasized the more emotional aspects of cooking. Jonas, for example, had a sign by the kitchen stove shouting 'Love!' When I asked about it he emphasized that 'Food is love.'

Thirdly, and perhaps somewhat contradictory, Johan's cooking philosophy also emerged as relatively accommodating. Even though concerned with healthy food, he was stricter with his own diet than that of his daughter and during the everyday stress he could be less strict. With some exceptions, despite their focus on health, the fathers in this group seemed rather permissive and pragmatic. Mikael, for example, underlined that ice cream was often an efficient part of the negotiations to get his two children (preschoolers) to eat vegetables. Most of the fathers cooked meals, but had no problem resorting to ready-made food like frozen pizzas, meatballs, lasagne or spring rolls if under time pressure or just tired—a convenience that is generally considered as being in opposition to "homely love" (Warde 1997, 132–133). This permissiveness offered pragmatic resistance to the intensive and self-sacrificing mothering ideology (Hays 1996) and instead followed a more pragmatic attitude to cooking—negotiating between ideals and what is practically possible (Carrigan and Szmigin 2006; Gram and Pedersen 2014). Overall, the fathers in this group were comfortable in their practice and did not express any worry about their way of handling it. With a few exceptions, they do not feel bad about resorting to easier solutions such as ready-made food every now and then.

Cooking as a hardship

Just a generation ago fathers appeared as all thumbs when it came to cooking. But while the group above presented an interest in food and cooking that with the professionalization and rising status of food safeguarded their masculinities (Neuman, Gottzén and Fjellström 2015; Parasecoli 2008), there was also a group of four that, in line with a more traditional masculinity (DeVault 1991; Lupton 1996), indicated that cooking was really not their thing. Magnus, for example, whose daughter Sara lived equally with both her parents after their divorce, explained how he had to come to terms with the fact that Sara preferred her grandmother's elk burgers to his relatively simple cooking: "Sara just has to go with the flow, and she appreciates her father anyway, so to speak."

But even if his cooking was simpler than his ex-wife's and mother-in-law's, Magnus stressed that he cared about making something for her that she both liked and was healthy. This particular evening he was serving sausages with rice and when I asked him if there would be any vegetables, he said probably grated carrots "or something." Contrary to the worry mothers can have concerning their cooking skills (Molander 2011), Magnus expressed none. While not a priority of his, he said he did as best as he could. Just like Johan, Magnus unconcernedly dealt with food based on his own interest and skill and focused on its value as a fuel.

This more permissive attitude towards cooking was also something the fathers indicated that their children gave voice to. Bo, a father of four (one preschooler and three teens), said his children accepted his bad cooking. He always made sure to have a bunch of standard dishes at home, be it "Willy's ready-made skewers with teriyaki sauce", "Willy's ready-made Thai box", "Willy's ready-made potato patties" or the ingredients for making pasta with avocado and blue cheese sauce. He said the kids were understanding:

> So they never make me feel bad [for my bad cooking], like 'dad, you really should' or 'when we're at mom's' because she's so much better at cooking. Never any comparison. They would never, ever make me feel bad about the fact that the meals [I prepare] aren't the most sophisticated and advanced.

Bo emphasized how happy he was for the good relationship he and his children had built up after the divorce. He stressed, however, that this fact did not stem from his cooking, but rather from their many conversations. Bo said he was more or less always around, usually sitting in the kitchen after work. And even though they seldom had any organized dinners together, one kid after the other could sit down and have a talk before running off to their next thing. While women often worry about, and are judged for, not caring enough (Doucet 2006) and where cooking is usually seen as a materialization of this care (Molander 2011), this was not what these fathers expressed. A low interest in cooking and bad cooking skills simply did not seem problematic for either Magnus or Bo.

The other two fathers in this group, however, did express something that seemed like concern. Dante, who had sole custody of his daughter of eight, underlined that cooking was something he needed to work on. He said his daughter was conservative and rarely appreciated anything other than spaghetti and meatballs with ketchup and he was worried she ate too many carbohydrates and not enough meat. In other words, just like the other fathers, his focus was on nourishment, on food as fuel. Still, Dante's parental priority seemed to be schoolwork rather than food. Three of his four diary photos by the kitchen table were of homework and only one of food—the breakfast.

Then there was Hans who had two (a grade-schooler and a teen) of his three children living with him half the time while his eldest had moved away from home. He did not compare himself to the children's mother, who was far from a star in the kitchen and who mostly bought expensive ready-made meals, but to his neighbor, another single father:

> When it comes to cooking, I don't really have it in me. It's a circus at our place and I haven't really prioritized food. // [But] I get a bit jealous of the neighbor, for example // I see him, he has like an apron on every evening and cooks, and I see how he sits down, I see that it's a ritual as well, he sits down and eats and discusses things with his children you know. And even if I cook, I don't feel like that // I'm not good at planning ahead, I plan pretty poorly and then all of a sudden I remember that 'Oh right, we're going to have dinner too' // So, I do a bit of a quick fix, just putting together whatever happens to be in the fridge.

As demonstrated in the quote above, Hans emerged as dissatisfied with the way he practiced cooking, not so much because of the nutritional deficiencies as the care that he seemed to think was lacking in his quick fix dinners. Rather than seeing food as fuel, to him food was more associated with the togetherness the meal made possible as well as the sacrifice of time needed to accomplish this; including the planning, the actual cooking and the continuity. He hereby expressed the same concerns as many mothers who worry about not sacrificing enough (Doucet 2006). Hans, who stayed at home with the children while their mother had a career, stuck out that way. Rather than the type of self-assurance and efficiency that many of the other fathers expressed in relation to dinner—a quick supply of fuel before running off to the next thing—Hans' thoughts about cooking were more in line with "traditional culinary femininities" (Szabo 2014) which includes not only cooking as love and care, but anxiety for not caring enough. Even if his years as a stay-at-home-dad in the private sphere obviously had not made him a better cook, it had made him experience the importance of routine parenting in everyday life at home as opposed to only filling the days with the children with exciting activities. He missed the daily routines after the divorce:

> I think [the children and I] should have [more of] this everyday life together that sometimes can be a bit annoying with homework, cleaning the car and the house and all the chores that need to be done. I want to be part of their everyday lives /.../ I struggle a lot with that.

In summary, the fathers in this group pointed out explicitly that their cooking abilities were not good but their perspective on it forked in two different directions. Magnus and Bo were pretty much unconcerned while Dante and Hans were bothered about it. Although they all resorted to easier solutions, Magnus and Bo considered it a fact of life, whereas Dante and Hans felt that they should make a greater effort, in other words sacrificing more (Cappellini and Parsons 2012)—no matter whether they did it to refuel or create togetherness.

Cooking as a part of life

> Well, I think, during the weekdays we often have quick dinners, because even when they aren't going off to workouts and practice, they often go out to meet friends and stuff ... Well, it's more during the weekends that you sit down and have dinner for a little longer.

Thomas, who had sole custody of three girls (two grade-schoolers and one teen) while working full time was part of the last group of four that was relatively disparate but had in common that none of them expressed an explicit interest in food or any difficulties related to it. They more or less spoke of it as an evident part of their daily lives as fathers. As Thomas' quote above illustrates, these fathers seemed to be in a constant rush. Things had to be done and done as efficiently as possible. They had some basic rules they stuck to but were relatively pragmatic. They simply did not spend time pondering about food, whether for themselves or for their children. Food was a fact, it had to be handled, and they were convinced that they did their best at handling it.

One of the basic rules was efficiency, a trait that is deeply associated with masculinity (Ross-Smith and Kornberger 2004). The fathers did not, for example, like throwing away food or time. Per, father of two boys (a pre-schooler and a teen), expressed his frustration over micro shopping; buying a little each day: "I'll try [online shopping]. I have to find another concept to minimize time waste." Thomas, in turn, saved time by shopping in-between dropping off and picking up the girls at their various activities. On Tuesdays, he had a gap of unused time when he took the opportunity to shop. When working late, he prepared lasagne, a leftover from the weekend, for the girls to put in the oven. Ulf, father of a boy and a girl (a grade-schooler and a teen), seemed less frustrated over wasting time but instead expressed frustration over wasting food and had therefore gone over to micro shopping together with his children more or less every day. Ulf underlined that the children had to learn to come to an agreement on what to eat during their shopping tours together to avoid wasting food, or else there would be no dinner.

A second basic rule was involving the children in some way. Like most of the fathers, Ulf and his children had dinner together most evenings during the weeks they lived together. In addition to shopping together with his sister, Ulf's son usually helped out with the cooking. As the family was usually busy with sports, shopping and cooking after work and school, dinners could be quite late. To Ulf that was simply a fact of life. Also Thomas, who had sole custody and worked full-time, had increasingly involved his girls in the cooking. His life seemed to circulate around work, household duties and driving the children between different activities. Even if the girls were busy with sports and school they were in charge of the food one day a week and could then cook whatever they liked.

Another basic rule in this group was, as Per called it, to be "reasonably observant" about healthy eating while still minimizing time loss. This meant they could not have fresh vegetables every day even if he would have liked to as it required shopping frequently. Ulf said that although he preferred home-cooked food to frozen pizza heated in the oven, it would never cross his mind to waste time on homemade meatballs—that was his limit for reasonable observance. Thomas, in turn, was concerned about his girls eating vegetables every day and tried to minimize the intake of junk food by never keeping it at home. But his reasonable observance included buying ready-made potato tots for his daughter who was vegetarian, ready-made fish sticks for the smallest daughter who he believed ate too little fish or giving the girls a hot dog in a bun when they were in a rush to get to their activities. Again, the men did not express concern over not sacrificing or caring enough (Lupton 1996), but appeared to be relatively pragmatic when negotiating between ideals and what was practically possible (Carrigan and Szmigin 2006; Gram and Pedersen 2014). With their focus on nourishment, their reasonable observance was also clearly related to the fact that they saw food as fuel.

In summary, to this group cooking did not stem from any specific interest or disinterest but was part of the daily flow of life and had to be handled, preferably according to some basic rules that included efficiency, involving the children and serving food that was reasonably healthy—a reasonable fuel.

Discussion

While research has shown Swedish men have a greater interest in taking responsibility for cooking (Neuman and Fjellström 2014) we still need to know more about how fathers experience and perform this consumption activity on an everyday basis, in particular those who combine work life and care in ways approaching the long held Swedish ideal of dual emancipation.

Contrary to the stigma experienced by the stay-at-home-fathers in Coskuner-Balli and Thompson's (2013) study, the cooking fathers in this study did not express any concern about emasculation. Instead, they saw it as self-evident to care for their children confirming that part of the ideal masculinity in Sweden today is indeed the caregiving father (Plantin 2015). Most of the fathers were also firmly anchored in their professional identities, one of the major building blocks of masculinity, and this seemed to counterbalance the stigma that stay-at-home fathers can face when engaging in care work (Doucet 2006). Half of the men in this study also expressed a great interest in cooking. Practicing fatherhood through cooking was self-evident to most of them and since it is steadily rising in the status hierarchy (Jönsson 2012) they could engage in it without running the risk of emasculation.

Furthermore, most of the fathers did not worry about whether their cooking was good enough or seek confirmation regarding any parental standard. While public institutions, various types of experts and others are trying to regulate motherhood and thereby create guilt and anxiety around the experience of mothering (See introduction of this volume; Lupton 1996; Rich 1986), this did not seem like a problem for these more easy going fathers who had already won "brownie points" by caring as much as they did through their joint or sole custody (Doucet 2006). Although they cared, the men appeared to have a more autonomous relationship with their children than women whose identity has been and is traditionally more anchored in being a mother. Also, expectations on them were already lower so most of the fathers had a low anxiety approach and were content with doing the best that they could.

No matter how they approached cooking, their relation to the market was generally relaxed and permissive, and they saw no problem in retreating to market solutions every now and then. Rather than turning to the market because they were concerned or even feared they did not make the grade in comparison to mothers (Doucet 2006; Molander 2011; Prothero 2006), these fathers seemed to turn to the market for pragmatic reasons—storing up on various types of ready-made meals for when they were in too much of a hurry, could not or simply did not want to cook. They merely juggled their professional and father identities as best they could and did not seem to worry about it.

However, and in line with recent research (Neuman, Gottzén and Fjellström 2015; Szabo 2014), instead of a strict division between traditional culinary masculinities and femininities, many times the men's masculinity-coded cooking mannerisms, such as efficiency and functionality, were mixed up with female-coded attributes like love and care (Molander 2011). In fact, even if most of them saw food as fuel and a means to an end rather than an end in itself, the type of childcare fathers are mostly associated with is highly related to this need for fuel, namely sports (Forsberg 2009; Gottzén, and Kremer-Sadlik 2012). According to Szabo (2014), discussions about men's emotions around food work are comparatively rare. This study contributes to this discussion by arguing for a reconsideration of the dichotomy between rationality and emotionality as the data exposed how blurred the lines actually are. Even if the fathers in their strive for efficiency appeared to be more functionally oriented and pragmatic in their dealings with food than mothers usually are depicted to be (see DeVault 1991; Lupton 1996; Molander 2011), there is no doubt that their cooking was an expression of love and care. It was just that their approach to caring differed from the self-effacing and sacrificing care that usually comes with motherhood (Cappellini and Parsons 2012; Hays 1996). The self-sacrifice and anxiety that Szabo (2014) also found among men who took a greater responsibility for cooking was, however, not found among the men in this study—to them convenience did not necessarily lead to less care (see Warde 1997). While on the one hand their caring was mixed with marketplace masculinity that includes competition, instrumentality and efficiency, it perhaps foremost reflected dual emancipation, prioritizing pragmatism over sacrifice—simply because there was no time for sacrifice when juggling between professional work and caring work. Indeed, even if rational and functionally oriented, the fathers' approach to food was also drenched with emotions displayed in the details, like the breakfast Björn served promptly at six o'clock every morning to make sure his son got plenty of nourishment: "Well, rather than just 'Oh shit, we're in a hurry. Eat your sandwich on the bus,' I mean, you just to get up [in time], you know, and make breakfast."

Whatever their approach to cooking they handled the situation matter-of-factly. They were pragmatic, did the best they could and saw it as good enough. While these men in many ways emerge as the vanguard for a new type of caring masculinity, the question is, whether we ought to hope for them to become the vanguard for a new type of parenting all together. Competition, instrumentality and efficiency aside, it could in fact be beneficial for society at large if these single fathers' more pragmatic relationship with the market, food, cooking and caring took hold among mothers whose caring today is often permeated by completely impossible demands. In short, let us hope new types of emancipated masculinities, comfortable in both private and public spheres, leads the way to a kind of caring that is not judged so harshly, by the parents themselves or by society at large.

References

Aarseth, H., and Olsen, B. M. (2008). Food and masculinity in dual-career couples. *Journal of Gender Studies*, 17(4): 277–287.

Bates, M. J., and Gentry, J. W. (1994). Keeping the family together: How we survived the divorce. *NA-Advances in Consumer Research*, 21.

Beck, U., and Beck-Gernsheim, E. (1995). *The Normal Chaos of Love*. Cambridge: Polity Press.

Bekkengen, L. (2003). Föräldralediga män och barnorienterad maskulinitet [Men on parental leave and child oriented masculinity]. In: T. Johansson and J. Kuosmanen, eds., *Manlighetens många ansikten: Fäder, feminister, frisörer och andra män* [The many faces of manliness: Fathers, feminists, hairdressers and other men]. Malmö: Liber, pp. 181–202.

Brandth, B. and Kvande, E. (eds.) (2013). *Fedrekvoten og den farsvennlige velferdsstaten*, [The parternal leave quota and the fatherhood friendly welfare state], Oslo, Norway: Universitetsforlaget.

Bugge, A. B., and Almås, R. (2006). Domestic dinner representations and practices of a proper meal among young suburban mothers. *Journal of Consumer Culture*, 6(2): 203–228.

Cappellini, B. and Parsons, E. (2012). (Re)enacting Motherhood: Self-sacrifice and Abnegation in the Kitchen. In: R.W. Belk and A. Ruvio, eds., *Identity and Consumption*, London: Routledge, pp. 119–128.

Carrigan, M., and Szmigin, I. (2006). Mothers of invention: Maternal empowerment and convenience consumption. *European journal of Marketing*, 40(9/10): 1122–1142.

Coskuner-Balli, G., and Thompson, C. J. (2013). The Status costs of subordinate cultural capital: At-home fathers' collective pursuit of cultural legitimacy through capitalizing consumption practices. *Journal of Consumer Research*, 40(1): 19–41.

DeVault, M. L. (1991). *Feeding the Family: The Social Organization of Caring as Gendered Work*. Chicago: University of Chicago Press.
Doucet, A. (2006). *Do men mother?: Fathering, Care, and Domestic Responsibility*. Toronto: University of Toronto Press.
Duvander, A-Z, Ferrarini, T., and Johansson, M. (2015). Familjepolitik för alla? En ESO-rapport om föräldrapenning och jämställdhetç [Family politics for all? An ESO report on parental leave and gender equality], *Rapport till Expertgruppen för studier i offentlig ekonomi*, 2015:5.
Ekström, M. P. (2016). Fler män lagar mat [More men are cooking], *CFK Nyheter* 2016-05-27.
Försäkringskassan (2013). De jämställda föräldrarna. Vad ökar sannolikheten för ett jämställt föräldrapenninguttag? [The equal parents. What increases the probability for an equal parental benefit withdrawal] *Socialförsäkringsrapport*, 8. Available at: www.forsakringskassan.se/wps/wcm/connect/8ec6c929-6f18-4e81-831f-cd4dbbaca 98e/socialforsakringsrapport_2013_08.pdf?MOD=AJPERES, [Accessed 20 November 2014].
Forsberg, L. (2009). *Involved parenthood. everyday lives of Swedish middle-class families*, Linköping Studies in Arts and Science No. 473.
Gentry, J., and Harrison, R. (2010). Is advertising a barrier to male movement toward gender change? *Marketing Theory*, 10(1): 74–96.
Gottzén, L., and Kremer-SadlikT. (2012). Expectations, fatherhood and youth sports: A balancing act between care and expectations. *Gender & Society*, 26(4): 639–664.
Gram, M., and Pedersen, H.D. (2014) Negotiations of Motherhood–between ideals and practice. In: S. O'Donohue, M. Hogg, P. Maclaran, L. Martens and L. Stevens, eds., *Motherhood, Markets and Consumption. The Making of Mothers in Contemporary Western Cultures*. London: Routledge, pp.56–67.
Harrison, R. L., Gentry, J. W., and CommuriS. (2012). A grounded theory of transition to involved parenting: The role of household production and consumption in the lives of single fathers. In: A.A. Ruvio and R. W. Belk, eds., *Gender, Culture, and Consumer Behavior*. London: Routledge, pp. 335–365.
Hays, S. (1996). *The Cultural Contradictions of Motherhood*. New Haven: Yale University Press.
Heisley, D. D., and Levy, S. J. (1991). Autodriving: A photoelicitation technique. *Journal of Consumer Research*, 18(3): 257–272.
Hochschild, A. (1989). *The second shift: Working parents and the revolution at home*. New York: Viking.
Holt, D. B., and ThompsonC. J. (2004). Man-of-action heroes: The pursuit of heroic masculinity in everyday consumption. *Journal of Consumer Research*, 31(2): 425–440.
Jönsson, H. (2012). *Den gastronomiska revolutionen* [The gastronomic revolution]. Stockholm: Carlsson Bokförlag.
Kimmel, M. S. (2012). *Manhood in America. A cultural history*. Oxford: Oxford University Press.
Kimmel, M. S. (2013). Masculinity as Homophobia: Fear, Shame, and Silence in the Construction of Gender Identity. In: M. M., Gergen and S. N. Davis eds., *Toward a New Psychology of Gender: A Reader*. New York: Routledge, pp. 223–242.
Klasson, M., and Ulver, S. (2015). Masculinising domesticity: An investigation of men's domestic foodwork. *Journal of Marketing Management*, 31(15–16): 1652–1675.

Klinth, R. (2002). *Göra pappa med barn: Den svenska pappapolitiken 1960–1995* [Making dad pregnant. The Swedish father politics. 1960–1995] Doctoral thesis. Linköping University.
Lupton, D. (1996). *Food, the body and the self.* London: Sage.
Marshall, D., Davies, T., Hogg, M., Schneider, T., and Petersen, A. 2014. "From Overt Provider to Invisible Presence: Discursive Shifts in Advertising Portrayals of the Father in Good Housekeeping, 1950–2010." *Journal of Marketing Management* 30 (15–16): 1654–1679.
Mellström, U. (2006). Nytt faderskap i skärningspunkten mellan produktion och reproduktion? [New fatherhood in the intersection between production and reproduction] *Socialvetenskaplig tidskrift*, 2:2006.
Miller, D. (1998). *A Theory of Shopping.* Oxford: Polity Press.
Moisio, R., Arnould, E.J., and PriceL.L. (2004). Between mothers and markets: Constructing family identity through homemade food. *Journal of Consumer Culture*, 4(3): 361–384.
Molander, S. (2011). *Mat, kärlek och metapraktik: En studie i vardagsmiddagskonsumtion bland ensamstående mödrar* [Food, love and meta-practices: A study in everyday dinner consumption among single mothers], Doctoral thesis. Stockholm: Företagsekonomiska institutionen, Stockholms universitet.
Neuman, N., and Fjellström, C. (2014). Gendered and gendering practices of food and cooking: An inquiry into authorisation, legitimisation and androcentric dividends in three social fields. *NORMA: International Journal for Masculinity Studies*, 9 (4): 269–285.
Neuman, N., Gottzén, L., and Fjellström, C. (2015). Narratives of progress: Cooking and gender equality among Swedish men. *Journal of Gender Studies*:1–13.
Östberg, J. (2012). Masculine Self-Presentation. In: A.A. Ruvio and R. W. Belk, eds., *Gender, Culture, and Consumer Behavior.* London: Routledge, pp. 129–136.
Parasecoli, F. (2008). *Bite me: Food in popular culture.* Oxford: Berg.
Plantin, L. (2003). Faderskap i retorik och praktik. Om 'nya' fäder i gamla strukturer [Fatherhood in rhetoric and practice. On 'new' fathers in old structures]. In: M. Bäck-Wiklund, and T. Johansson, eds., *Nätverksfamiljen* [The network family]. Stockholm: Natur och kultur, pp. 143–159.
Plantin, L. (2015). Contemporary Fatherhood in Sweden: Fathering Across Work and Family Life. In: J. L. Roopnarine, eds., *Fathers Across Cultures. The Importance, Roles and Diverse Practices of Dads.* Santa Barbara, California: ABC-CLIO, pp. 91–107.
Prothero, A. (2006). The F-word: The use of fear in advertising to mothers. *Advertising & Society Review*, 7(4).
Rich, A. (1986). *Of Woman Born: Motherhood as Experience and Institution.* New York: WW Norton.
Robinson, B. K., and Hunter, E. (2008). Is mom still doing it all? Reexamining depictions of family work in popular advertising. *Journal of Family Issues*, 29(4): 465–486.
Ross-Smith, A., and Kornberger, M. (2004). Gendered rationality? A genealogical exploration of the philosophical and sociological conceptions of rationality, masculinity, and organization. *Gender, Work, and Organization*, 11(3): 280–305.
SCB (2010). Tidsanvändningsundersökningen 2010 [The time usage study 2012]. [online]. Available at: www.scb.se/Pages/PressRelease___319925.aspx. [Accessed 4 April 2013].

SCB (2014). Olika familjer lever på olika sätta—om barns boende och försörjning efter en separation. *Demografiska rapporter*, 1. [online]. Available at: www.scb.se/Statistik/_Publikationer/BE0701_2013A01_BR_BE51BR1401.pdf [Accessed 17 November 2014].
Spicer, A. and Cederström, C. (2015). *Wellnessyndromet* [The wellness syndrome]. Stockholm: Tankekraft förlag.
Szabo, M. (2013). Foodwork or foodplay? Men's domestic cooking, privilege and leisure. *Sociology*, 47(4): 623–638.
Szabo, M. (2014). Men nurturing through food: Challenging gender dichotomies around domestic cooking. *Journal of Gender Studies*, 23(1): 18–31.
Thompson, C. J., Locander, W. B., and Pollio, H.R. (1989). Putting consumer experience back into consumer research: The philosophy and method of existential-phenomenology. *Journal of Consumer Research*, 16(2): 133–146.
Tinson, J., Nancarrow, C., and Brace, I. (2008). Purchase decision making and the increasing significance of family types. *Journal of Consumer Marketing*, 25(1): 45–56.
Warde, A. (1997). *Consumption, Food and Taste*. London: Sage.
Wilk, R. (2010). Power at the table: Food fights and happy meals. *Cultural Studies: Critical Methodologies*, 10(6): 428–436.
World Economic Forum (2014). The Global Gender Gap Report 2014, [online]. Available at http://reports.weforum.org/global-gender-gap-report-2014/ [Accessed 19 October 2016].

Chapter 11

Calibrating motherhood

Kate Cairns, Josée Johnston and Merin Oleschuk

Introduction

It is not difficult to conjure the image of a "bad mom" feeding her child "bad food". This is the woman with a shopping cart full of soda and processed junk, who sends her kids to school with unhealthy snacks, and who is charged with raising obese children. These images abound in popular culture, and connect to a substantive literature on mother blame (Boero 2010; Ladd-Taylor & Umansky 1998). Scholars rightly emphasize how stigmatized images such as these work to shame women for domestic foodwork – particularly poor or working-class women and women of color– and reveal how marginalized mothers struggle to feed their children under surveillance from state authorities (Elliott et al. 2016; Wright, Maher & Tanner 2015). While this form of the "bad" mom has become a familiar figure in media and academic discourse, in this chapter we investigate its presence alongside a second stigmatized version of mothering: namely, the mom who obsesses over feeding her children only the healthiest, purest, "good" food. This overbearing mother constantly guards her brood from the dangers of transfats, pesticides, and non-organic milk, and is connected to stereotypes of thin, white, upper-middle class motherhood. Paranoid about the dangers of processed foods, this mother forbids her kids from eating cake at a birthday party, and instead offers up mealy homemade cookies and gluten-free snacks that few children could genuinely enjoy.

While this depiction of the overbearing health-obsessed mother is clearly an exaggerated portrayal, we argue that this imagined figure serves an important purpose in contemporary food discourse: to police the boundaries of acceptable maternal foodwork. Just as the uninformed "McDonald's Mom" has been deemed unacceptable, the neurotic "Organic Mom" is also stigmatized, albeit with considerably less social penalty given the privilege associated with this position. While feeding children, mothers must work to distance themselves from both extremes, a process that we call *calibration* (Cairns & Johnston 2015a). Through calibration, mothers separate themselves from two opposing figures: the uninformed or uncaring "bad mom," but also, the overly invested, controlling "perfect Mom" who cares too much and appears obsessive. In the realm of feeding children, the performance of maternal femininity involves the ongoing negotiation of identities and food practices to avoid the appearance of caring too little, or too much, about children's food practices.

In this chapter, we explore these two maternal figures as they manifest in mothers' feeding narratives. Before delving into our analysis, we outline feminist scholarship on the penalties of maternal foodwork, and point to the emergence of the overbearing food-obsessed mother as a recent empirical and conceptual development. We explore how these two maternal figures manifest in interviews and focus groups with Canadian mothers, with a focus on mothers' ongoing calibration to distance themselves from stigmatized extremes. We close with a brief discussion of the raced and classed implications of these two maternal figures as well as their relationship to contemporary childhood ideals.

Feminist approaches to maternal foodwork

Feminist scholarship reveals a long-established connection between successful foodwork, femininity and good mothering (Lupton 1996; Charles & Kerr 1988; Bugge & Almas 2006). As Marjorie DeVault famously stated, caring for others through food is central to the performance of maternal femininities, allowing mothers to present themselves as "recognizably womanly" (1991, p. 118). The "good mother" is idealized as one who provides nutritious, yet delicious, homemade meals and teaches children to make healthy food choices. The cultural exaltation of the good mother brings harsh scrutiny and judgment toward those who are seen to fail in this performance, whether by serving overly processed foods, or raising children with an unacceptable level of body fat (Boero 2010; Herndon 2010; Warin et al. 2012). This judgment is particular (though not exclusive) to women. While men are taking up foodwork in increasing numbers, with some becoming active in home cooking (Szabo 2014), it remains clear that most of the work of feeding children continues to be coded feminine and carried out by women (Bianchi et al. 2000; Cairns & Johnston 2015a; Sayer 2005). Good mothers may have help from a partner, but continue to do most of the domestic foodwork involving children. This inequitable domestic burden is justified in various ways: women are seen to be "naturally" more interested in food, children's health, and maintaining high food standards, and may seek to avoid conflict over foodwork (Beagan et al. 2008). In the words of one Canadian mother, "it's just easier for me to do it" (ibid).

Defined by her capacity to nurture and socialize the next generation, the good mother is constructed in relation to the figure of the child (Cook 2009). Mothers are seen to be uniquely attuned to children's needs, and personally responsible for ensuring their physical, intellectual and social development

(Burman & Stacey 2010). Put simply, maternal foodwork is fundamentally constituted by shared understandings of childhood, and these understandings are historically and culturally specific (Lupton 2014). In North America, a key aspect of contemporary maternal foodwork involves managing the industrial food risks thought to threaten children's health (MacKendrick 2014; MacKendrick & Stevens 2016). Accordingly, the good mother strives to raise an "organic child" who is shielded from pesticides, added hormones, or other industrial contaminants, and socialized to make ethical food choices (Cairns, Johnston & MacKendrick 2013). These feeding standards position children as pure beings in need of protection (Murphy 2000), and dovetail with an intensive mothering ideology that defines successful childrearing as a selfless project involving endless research, investment, and emotional labor (Hays 1996; Cairns & Johnston 2015a, p. 69). The organic child ideal is especially penalizing for poor and working-class mothers, given the substantial economic and cultural capital required to even approximate such intensive feeding practices, as well as the privileged class associations of "alternative" foods (Cairns, Johnston & MacKendrick 2013; Paddock 2015; Johnston & Baumann 2015). Some standards of maternal foodwork resonate across class, including the importance of providing access to healthy foods, like fruits and vegetables (Beagan et al. 2014; Wright, Maher & Tanner 2015). Yet mothers' access to and understanding of "good" and "bad" foods also varies across class contexts, reflecting and reinforcing classed-based inequalities (Wright, Maher & Tanner 2015). Additionally, many of these foodwork ideals are difficult to achieve on a limited income, such as introducing children to a diversity of new foods (Daniel 2016).

Our research shows that even when mothers are critical of the gendered pressures surrounding foodwork, the emotional pull of mothering standards are difficult to dismiss (Cairns & Johnston 2015a, p. 67). It is one thing for a mother to recognize that women are judged harshly for their foodwork, but it is quite another for her to simply ignore collective feeding standards, especially given the common desire to provide the very best for one's children (see Webster, this volume). Women derive emotional rewards from approximating the organic child ideal, and risk social judgment when they eschew these standards, or lack the resources required to pursue them. Put in different terms, women actively work to avoid the stigma of being a "bad" mother who feeds her children "bad" food, understanding stigma in the Goffmanian sense of being a "deeply discrediting" attribute or mark that shifts one from being a normal, respectable person to a "tainted discounted one" (Goffman 1963, p. 3). Stigmas are sociologically significant because they work to disadvantage certain groups, enable discrimination, and link people to harmful stereotypes (Link & Phelan 2001, p. 365).

Scholars have analyzed the stigmatized identity associated with "bad" feeding practices often ascribed to a poor or working-class mother who is said to lack knowledge and self-control (Boero 2010; Herndon 2010). Below, we refer to this imagined figure as the "McDonald's Mom," given mothers' frequent references to the fast food chain during interviews and focus groups. As mothers in our study distanced themselves from an unhealthy "Other" who made poor food choices, McDonald's seemed to function as a trope symbolizing "easy" meals, "unhealthy" choices, and "bad" mothering more generally. Less scholarly attention has been given to the stigma associated with the opposite extreme of "good" feeding – the controlling upper-middle-class mother, whom we can think about as the overbearing "Organic Mom". Our conversations with women highlight the existence of not one, but *two* pathologized poles – the inattentive mother who makes poor choices and relies on processed foods and the controlling mother who obsessively monitors and manages her child's diet. We argue that these two figures enter into maternal foodwork through the process of calibration, as mothers work to distance their own feeding practices from each pathologized extreme (Cairns & Johnston 2015a). More than simply staking a "safe" middle ground, calibration involves an ongoing negotiation of food identities and practices so as to avoid the impression of obsessive control on the one hand, and irresponsible indulgence on the other.

Certainly these two stigmatized figures do not entail equal amounts of social sanction. The stigma of being perceived as a lazy, ignorant "bad" feeder is likely to be much more socially discrediting given its connection to classed and racist stereotypes (Boero 2010; Bowen, Elliott, & Brenton 2014; Wright, Maher & Tanner 2015), and thus to engender significantly more discrimination and surveillance – including surveillance from state authorities (Elliott et al. 2016; Wright, Maher & Tanner 2015). What's more, an individual woman's relationship to these imagined figures is shaped by her social location. Because of the classed and racialized stereotypes associated with "good" and "bad" feeding practices (Boero 2010; Elliott et al. 2016), the threat of being categorized as a "McDonald's Mom" is clearly greater for poor women and women of color than for affluent white women. Our point here is that the presence of stigma at both foodwork extremes suggests a gendered process wherein the performance of "acceptable" motherhood requires a constant balancing act. Put differently, women must continually monitor and manage their children's food consumption in ways that are careful and responsible, yet don't appear obsessive and overly controlling. We stress that this process is labour-intensive and emotionally taxing, yet also endless; calibration involves a constant process of positioning within the performance of maternal food femininities. In the next section, we examine both poles of pathologized maternal foodwork as they manifest in women's feeding narratives.

Calibrating motherhood: interview and focus group narratives

Our analysis combines data from qualitative interviews and focus groups conducted with Toronto mothers as part of a broader study investigating the relationship between food and femininity (Cairns & Johnston 2015a). In this chapter, we draw from 10 interviews and 10 focus groups, for a combined total of 47 mothers. Our sample included 27 middle-class women and 20 working-class or poor women; the racial composition included 32 white women and 15 women of color. One participant was married to a woman, while all others were either single or partnered with men. The women engaged in a wide-variety of paid and unpaid work, and we use their own labels below to describe their work or occupational status. Although our sample was relatively diverse, it is important to note that our call for participants solicited participation from mothers who were interested in discussing food and foodwork, and this undoubtedly influenced our sample. (For more information on the study, see Cairns and Johnston 2015a, p. 14–18). During interviews and focus groups, we asked mothers about the priorities guiding their feeding practices, as well as any tensions they experienced in daily foodwork. Below, we turn our attention, first, to the role of the "McDonald's Mom" as she emerged in our data, and then to the opposing figure of the "Organic Mom".

The inattentive "McDonald's Mom"

During interviews and focus groups, mothers actively distanced themselves from a negative maternal figure that we call the "McDonald's Mom". These conversations were replete with concern about the deleterious impact of feeding children a steady diet of fast food and processed "junk". While such negative assessments were not limited to a single fast-food chain, we were struck by the ubiquity of references to McDonald's, in particular. Consistently positioned as a symbol of failed maternal foodwork, McDonald's came to stand in for quick, "easy" meals and unhealthy choices. For example, when discussing the importance of planning for healthy, home-cooked meals, Gail (white, acupuncturist) contrasted this vision with a "stereotypical image of someone stopping at McDonald's to get food for their kids on the way to soccer practice." Marissa (Black, project manager) confessed that as "busy people we do need to do fast food," but clarified that "my kids will tell you that does *not* mean McDonald's." Emphasizing the value of good food for physical and mental well-being, Marissa prioritized shared family meals and said that "going into McDonald's for your burger and sitting and sharing that greasy [food] – that's not going to do it." Carol (white, film producer) associated McDonald's with a sense of melancholy and fatigue, and expressed her goal of "trying to eat to stay happy ... and not go to McDonald's because you're too tired and depressed." Theresa (mixed race, unemployed/social assistance) described her extensive efforts to keep processed food out of the house, recalling how her son "went to a birthday party at McDonald's, came home and threw up because he just wasn't used to that food." Clearly proud of this anecdote, Theresa saw her son's intolerance for fast food as confirmation of her own devoted feeding work. Seen as a quick and unhealthy alternative to the home-cooked family meal, McDonald's connotes a maternal figure with insufficient knowledge, effort and attention to children's physical and social development.

Mothers in our study displayed a clear mental image of a mother who performs foodwork poorly, and sought to distance their own feeding practices from this figure. The imagined figure of the McDonald's Mom feeds her children fast food, relies on pre-packaged snacks, and is observed with a shopping cart full of "junk" at the grocery store. The failure of the McDonald's Mom is embodied in the child who prefers "junk" to nutritious meals, and is unable to identify vegetables or distinguish a pudding cup from a healthy yoghurt snack. To avoid the stigma associated with the McDonald's Mom, the "good" mother must make homemade meals, avoid the temptation of unhealthy shortcuts, and teach her children to appreciate and seek out "good" food. Thus, the McDonald's Mom operates as a stigmatized Other that mothers use to defend their own feeding practices. While this defense may seem judgmental at times, we suggest that mothers' efforts to establish distance from the McDonald's Mom reflect the intense pressure and scrutiny they experience in the everyday work of feeding children, and the perceived risk of resembling this figure at any moment.

The key traits of the McDonald's Mom were particularly evident in mothers' discussions of packed lunches. During focus groups, mothers commiserated over the challenge of packing a homemade lunch that their children would actually eat (and hopefully enjoy), and suggested that this project was made all the more difficult by the unhealthy feeding practices of others. As Brenda (white, stay-at-home mom) put it, "it's shocking what's in some of the kids' lunch bags. It really is." Similarly, Deb (Indigenous, unemployed/social assistance) described feeling "really shocked" by "what parents pack for their kids," and recalled fieldtrips when "kids come around to look at our lunches and they can't identify the vegetables." Mothers frequently described the challenge of sending children to school with a healthy, homemade meal that would not be traded for junk food. Tara (white, not working due to chronic pain, social assistance) shared that when her son was younger, "his friends would have these Fruit Roll-ups and like, all this crap." However, she expressed pride that, "as he got older I could talk to him about why I made these decisions and now he can understand and he's cool with it." In these discussions, it became clear that the maternal feeding work of the packed lunch goes beyond simply sending healthy food to school; mothers also engage in the laborious task of teaching children to navigate a food environment filled with "crap", and socializing them to make healthy food choices. In this socialization project, the McDonald's Mom not only serves as the failed Other, but also threatens to undermine mothers' feeding practices by populating children's social worlds with appealing, unhealthy alternatives.

While mothers' stories about the "junk" in other children's lunches drew clear "us and them" distinctions between good and bad feeding practices, the boundaries drawn around maternal foodwork were often complex and reflexive. Some women reflected critically on the challenge of producing "good" food, and of avoiding the McDonald's Mom in ones' own family foodwork. Struggling to maintain her high standards in the midst of her teenagers' love for processed foods, Sadie (white, cafeteria supervisor) said, "I don't want to just abandon all hope and buy Aunt Jemima pancake mix ... I do want to keep a dialogue going." Other women identified specific instances where they had behaved as the McDonald's Mom in the past. For example, Deirdre (white, farmers market manager) recalled making a video of her then-two-year-old daughter trying to say "Coca Cola" (which Deidre was drinking at the time) during a meal of ramen noodles and frozen vegetables. She described the discomfort she felt sharing this video with friends as it revealed her reliance on processed foods:

> I was ashamed to show them the ramen noodles and the frozen vegetables that she was eating. And whoever I was showing it to was like, "What are you feeding your kid?" .... I realized that I had some shame issues about what my kid was eating.

Deirdre framed this as a transformative moment within her own food narrative, a turning point in a longer shift that led her to local, seasonal, cooking from scratch. Reflecting on this transition, she described how her feelings toward foodwork changed from shame and embarrassment, to pride and joy; she worked to not only change the family's eating practices but also to teach her children about the sources of good food: "I'm so PROUD of the food that I've [provided] for my family. And that I know who grew it and where it came from."

While Deirdre positioned the McDonald's Mom safely behind her, many mothers expressed a more contested relationship to this figure. Far from a static accomplishment, the work of distancing oneself from stigmatized feeding practices is an ongoing process, changing as children age, standards shift, and life-circumstances evolve. This processual aspect of calibration was clear in Tammy's (white, daycare worker) story, as she described continuing negotiations with her husband, who eats "junk" food that Tammy sees as a threat to their child's health:

> I don't want [our son] to have the same eating habits that both of us and specifically my husband has. He drinks two litres of pop a day and eats specifically only white bread. He doesn't eat whole grain products at all. And it's getting to the point now where like, I'm asking him not to bring white bread into the house because I don't really want [our son] eating it.

Tammy's frustration with her husband's food choices illustrates the challenge of securing the "good" mother performance. Despite her best efforts to shield her son from the perils of processed foods, these very foods are entering her home – and she feels personally responsible for limiting her child's access to them. In other cases, mothers described the challenge of promoting healthy feeding practices as children grew older and gained greater autonomy over their food choices. Sadie's sons had been raised on a vegetarian diet of home-cooked meals, but later joined their friends in purchasing hamburgers made of "hyper-industrialized processed beef." She shared the story of a birthday party when she had purchased "sparkling organic juice" as a special treat only to learn that her son "snuck off with his friends and bought a big thing of Coke". No matter the level of maternal devotion, it was clear in our research that achieving distance from the McDonald's Mom was an ongoing challenge that generated frustration and guilt for mothers.

The process of avoiding this stigmatized maternal figure is not straightforwardly about isolating kids from junk food, but also involves health education. The McDonald's Mom is a failed educator; she does not teach her children how to moderate their treats, understand healthy choices, or try new foods. To distance herself from this stigmatized position, the good mother allows children the occasional treat, but trains them to exercise self-discipline. In Cindy's (white, fitness trainer) words, "I want them to be able to have the store-bought cookies, have two, put them away and not eat the entire row." Similarly, Gail (white acupuncturist) described efforts to help her son recognize the impact of junk food on his body:

> with things like sugar, trying to teach him that yeah it tastes really good in your mouth but later on your tummy feels bad if you have too much ... yeah, just allowing him some exposure to it but also teaching him how to use it well.

To not be positioned as the McDonald's Mom, mothers felt they must raise informed consumers who learn to resist junk food on their own. Indeed, mothers sometimes pointed toward children's good eating habits as evidence of their successful socialization efforts. For example, Carol (white, film producer) said, "I'm quite proud that my kids like to eat lots of good things. I like that they're not picky eaters." Similarly, Shannon (white, social assistance) noted that her teenage daughter "will eat pretty much anything. Since she was a toddler, we fed her whatever we were eating so that she wouldn't be a picky eater." Once children have knowledge about "good" food, they are then expected to one day choose and prepare good food for themselves. Alejandra (Hispanic, journalist) described an earnest desire for her daughter "to be able to say 'now [my parents] gave me the skills to learn how to cook and clean and take care of myself too,'" and added, "I don't think parents are doing their kids any favors by not teaching them those things." This image of the good mom who teaches her children how to cook was contrasted with the implied McDonald's Mom whose children don't know how to "boil water" or are "not allowed to go near the oven."

Throughout this section, we have shown how mothers from diverse class backgrounds engaged in boundary work to distinguish their feeding practices from the stigmatized figure of the McDonald's Mom, a common target for ridicule in contemporary food discourse. While these narratives emphasize mothers' successes in opposition to a failed Other, we do not want to imply that women in our study felt completely assured in their feeding practices; this is far from the truth. While expressing commitments to providing home-cooked, non-processed, nutritious meals and teaching their children to make healthy choices, mothers shared a range of worries and perceived failures that we have discussed elsewhere (Cairns, Johnston & MacKendrick 2013, Cairns et al. 2014, Cairns & Johnston 2015a), and are documented by other scholars (O'Connell & Brannen 2016; Wright, Maher & Tanner 2015). From concerns about children's exposure to harmful chemicals, to feelings of defeat in the face of a picky eater, to the endless frustration of trying to make nutritious choices on a limited income, the everyday work of feeding children is a realm of emotional labor, self-doubt, and interpersonal struggle. In fact, we see mothers' consistent and emphatic disapproval of the McDonald's Mom not as a sign of unflagging self-confidence, but rather, as a reflection of the acute gendered pressures associated with foodwork, and the resulting insecurities many mothers experience in their feeding practices. It is worth noting that a comparable figure of the "McDonald's Dad" did not emerge in our broader research (which included conversations with both men and women), a finding that reflects the more flexible, forgiving and capacious standards at play when men engage in social reproductive labor.

The overbearing "Organic Mom"

Distancing oneself from the negative extreme of the McDonald's Mom is a key component of the calibration process, but it is only half the story. In their rejection of fast food and their commitment to healthy, home-cooked meals, mothers risk resembling another stigmatized figure: the overly-invested and overbearing Organic Mom whose intensive feeding practices venture into the realm of excess. In this section we sketch out this pathologized figure who is located at the opposite extreme of maternal femininity, and implicitly coded as white and affluent. Think here of the heavily-involved mother who obsessively watches what her children eat, making sure all choices are nutritious and organic, homemade and local. Following MacKendrick and Pristavec (2016), we label this figure the "Organic Mom". The Organic Mom performs foodwork according to idealized maternal standards, but it is precisely her competency and commitment that generates stigma. She does the right thing, but she is uptight, controlling, and "crazy" while doing it. As feminist psychoanalytic and post-structuralist authors have theorized, the feminine figure is commonly constituted as the unhinged, irrational, "negatively signified Other" positioned in relation to the rational, clear-thinking man (e.g., Chesler 1974; Malson 1998, p. 32). Like the McDonald's Mom, the Organic Mom is not a "real" person, embodied in a singular mother's everyday foodwork. Rather, the Organic Mom functions as an imagined figure that women use to position their own feeding practices within a performance of daily maternal foodwork that is informed and dedicated, but not obsessively so.

In the contemporary North American story of good mothering, choosing organic foods for children is an idealized marker of maternal commitment (Cairns et al. 2013). Just as McDonald's serves as a symbol of unhealthy processed food, organics serve as a symbol of "pure" healthy foods that are safe for children to eat. Associated feeding practices go beyond certified organic products to include a range of foods understood to be "natural", unprocessed, or free from the chemical taint of industrialized foods. In line with the ideal of a pure, organic diet, mothers in our study with sufficient economic resources frequently referred to the Environmental Working Group's "Dirty Dozen" list of the most pesticide-laden fruits and vegetables as a key source of guidance. They also expressed a commitment to purchasing organic, or naturally-raised animal products for their children. Describing her meat-buying habits for her family, Carol (white, film producer) said, "I go to our butcher where it's all sort of grass-fed and raised. I'm weirded out by gross meat".

While our interviews and focus groups revealed clear maternal standards for "pure" foods that were deemed safe for developing children, we noticed a consistent pattern: when expressing their preference for these standards, mothers were careful to note that they were not overly concerned or dogmatic in their commitment. Put simply, mothers distanced themselves from the figure of the Organic Mom who is obsessive, militant, and inflexible in her feeding preferences. For example, Eva (white, nonprofit sector) said that she prioritized organic foods for her daughter, but clarified that "we're not anal about it." She added, "if [my daughter] is at my mom's house and my mom doesn't have anything organic or whatever it's just not a big deal." Like many women in our study, Selena (white, midwife) reported that, "anything that's in the top ten [of the Dirty Dozen list] for pesticides I try to buy organic, but sometimes I'm flexible." Carol also described following the "dirty list", but clarified that this was not a dogmatic devotion where she was duped into naïve overspending patterns: "Why bother buying organic when it's not sprayed to begin with? So, I don't buy organic broccoli. It's way down on the bottom [of the list]. But I buy organic berries."

What sets the Organic Mom apart is not simply her "pure" food purchases, but the dogmatism of her feeding ideals. We were struck by how many mothers distinguished their food practices from a form of maternal food "militancy". While Anne (white, stay-at-home mom) was clear that her kids are not fed certain foods like hotdogs, she also insisted, "I am not militant about it." Similarly, Tammy (white, daycare worker) explained that while she and her husband provide their son with healthy foods, they "try very hard also not to get into that urban, crunchy granola mafia kind of mindset." Elaine (Asian, research analyst) described how she "goes with the flow" when feeding her infant daughter, and contrasted this approach with friends who are "very militant about it ... it's almost as if it's a religion." Fran (white/Creole, administrative assistant) made a similar distinction, distancing her personal views on healthy eating from a militant Organic Mom who tries to indoctrinate others with her beliefs:

> I'm not militant in that sense where I don't feel it's a personal crusade to change everyone's dietary habits. It's very personal. Food is very, very personal, it's very cultural ... I don't feel it's my place to make that decision for anyone else.

The Organic Mom's dogmatism can lead her to become a crazed figure, obsessively pursuing pure standards at the expense of her mental health and social relationships. Like other women in our study, Lucia (Hispanic, social worker) prioritized organic meat for her family, but was clear that she did not allow these choices to become a source of anxiety: "What's the difference between organic and non-organic? ... I'm not going to stress my mind or my life about that." Similarly, Nancy (white, teacher) reported that while she has clear food standards, she maintains a relaxed kindness towards her shopping: "[I] tend to prefer organic, I tend to prefer fair trade ... I prefer nutritious food. So I have all these preferences but I let myself off the hook generally". Robin (white, student) said she prioritized organic milk for her kids, but was careful to qualify this preference, noting that she did not take these choices to ridiculous – or rude – extremes: "I'll still buy a regular thing of milk. I'm not going to be that picky about it ... [if we] go over to somebody's house for dinner, what's gracious is just, you know, you go and you eat it." In contrast to an image of obsessive maternal oversight, Robin described how she concedes control to others who are doing the foodwork, and thus avoids the perceived rudeness of the Organic Mom:

> if your grandparents want to stuff him full of licorice then I can't do much about it [laughter] ... I just feel like, this is our home and this is what we do in our home. And outside of our home is a whole big wide world, and hopefully what you do is you create good habits and send them on their way.

Besides rigidity and dogmatism, another key feature of the Organic Mom is her zealous pursuit of health and labelling schemes at the expense of her children's pleasure. Distancing themselves from this figure, mothers emphasized their efforts to balance health commitments with an appreciation for children's preferences and the importance of tasty treats. For example, after a lengthy discussion of Fran's detailed label reading routines (which involved elaborate strategies for considering organic content alongside salt levels, sugar content, fiber, and serving size), she emphasized that her concern for health did not lead her to dismiss culinary pleasure:

> I'm of the mindset, moderation is key ... There's times when we'll go out to a restaurant or we go out to a café for brunch. I know in all likelihood the ingredients are likely not local, they're not free range, they're not organic. ... But it's moderation. We don't do it all the time. It's a treat.

In keeping with this emphasis on moderation, many mothers insisted that their healthy feeding practices did not deny the "treats" of childhood. Eva (white, nonprofit sector) made clear that her daughter was not deprived, even though health was a priority in her foodwork:

> She still has Nutella every morning. [laughs] And I know it's not healthy, but what does she have it on? A whole grain pita. Along with her yogurt smoothie with organic yogurt and fruit. So it's not like we're depriving her.

While the controlling Organic Mom denies her child food pleasures, Eva insists that a chocolate hazelnut spread can be balanced with whole grains and an organic smoothie. Referring to the dinner her daughter was eating during our interview, Eva said that an "organic egg" balances out a treat so that, "now she can have chocolate if she wants".

Allowing a certain amount of "treats" appears central to avoiding the rigidity of the Organic Mom – even treats from McDonald's. Carol's (white, film producer) commitment to healthy, organic foodwork was notable in our sample, but she was careful to clarify that her kids still enjoy occasional treats like hamburgers, organic hotdogs, and nachos prepared at home, qualifying that it's "all done by hand". She also shared that her kids had even experienced the treats on offer at McDonald's:

> my daughter's five and we've been to McDonald's ten times on the road. Off the highway or something like that. So it's not that we completely always avoid it. .... You know, you can have a treat once in a while, there's nothing wrong with it.

Carol's emphasis on her children's access to a rare McDonald's "treat" reveals the complexity of the calibration process. While taking children to McDonald's is a hallmark of "bad" mothering practices, *total* rejection of this experience is also stigmatized. At this end of the spectrum sits the Organic Mom, whose rigid feeding practices prevent children from experiencing the quintessential treats of childhood. Achieving a "moderate" position between these two stigmatized extremes requires endless calibration, as well as the cultural and economic capital to precisely moderate children's exposure to "junky" treats.

In this section, we have argued that women engage in boundary work to demarcate their flexible, moderate foodwork from the stigmatized Organic Mom. Mothers frequently distanced themselves from this figure – an overwrought, pleasure-denying puritan who can't enjoy a treat. At the same time, we want to emphasize that this calibration was an active, ongoing process that often involved feelings of self-doubt. Just as women reflected on the presence of McDonald's Mom traits in their own behavior, women in our study also identified instances where they had behaved like the Organic Mom. For instance, Lisa said that while she now brings a more relaxed attitude to purchasing organic foods for her kids, she had taken a "more hard core" approach to feeding when they were younger. Reflecting on how mothers can "kind of get caught up in these things," she described her present-day practices as "not as hard core" as in the past, and juxtaposed her more relaxed current self against the rigidity of the Organic Mom.

Maternal calibration is clearly shaped by the intense threat of social judgment mothers encounter in their daily feeding practices. While women actively worked to manage the stigma associated with the McDonald's Mom and Organic Mom, they sometimes critiqued these very expectations. For example, Matilda (white, mediator) expressed frustration with what she called "all the shoulds" surrounding maternal foodwork, and said "sometimes I feel that's oppressive." This idea resonated with her friend Grace (white, management consultant), who added "it's enough to just make you say, damn this, I'm buying this anyway." As the discussion continued, this group of friends challenged the notion that the McDonald's Mom and the Organic Mom were static figures embodied by very different kinds of women; instead they situated these figures on a continuum of maternal foodwork and suggested that individual mothers regularly moved between them in the context of daily feeding practices. In Zahra's (South Asian, writer) words, "it depends on where you are, what your head space is, what your day is like. You know, is that the day you go to the [high-end organic store] or is that the day you go to the [discount supermarket]. Like, each thing is different." Laughing, Grace added, "Or is it the day I take the kids to McDonald's for a shake and French fries 'cause that way I won't kill them!" While Grace's comment was clearly meant as a joke, this discussion is illuminating. These women understood calibration to be an ongoing process in which the performance of the good mother remained elusive. Depending on the particular constraints of grocery budgets, scheduling, social relations, and emotional energy, mothers' feeding practices may resemble McDonald's Mom one day and Organic Mom the next. This is especially the case for mothers with ample economic and cultural capital, whose occasional trip to McDonald's is unlikely to garner social stigma. By contrast, poor mothers and mothers of color are rarely afforded such flexibility, and thus face greater risk of being aligned with this failed maternal figure.

Discussion and conclusion

Calibration involves a continual process of avoiding stigmatized extremes. In our interviews and focus groups, mothers worked to present their feeding practices as informed, but not dogmatic; they were committed, but not obsessed. This endless positioning speaks to the penalizing standards surrounding maternal foodwork – whether in the stigma of the uninformed, uncaring "McDonald's Mom," or the stigma of the uptight, annoying "Organic Mom". In addition, we find instances where the calibration process involves an element of critique, as mothers challenge penalizing standards of maternal femininity. While calibration was often expressed by exerting distance from an abject Other, we also saw instances where a commitment to more "flexible" standards allowed mothers to maintain a sense of dignity in their feeding work. Thus, we find that the calibration process has the potential to both affirm and challenge the McDonald's Mom and Organic Mom tropes. Women are not just cultural dupes in this process; they are reflexively critiquing and negotiating these standards in their everyday feeding practices.

While our analysis has primarily focused on gender, it is important to recognize that mothers' calibration efforts are shaped by relations of race and class (see Harman and Cappellini, this volume). The McDonald's Mom and the Organic Mom are clearly classed figures, with the perfectionist, controlling image of the latter signaling a particular upper-middle classed version of motherhood, and the McDonald's Mom associated with stereotypical images of an inattentive working-class or poor mother. These figures also have racialized dimensions, given the association between "alternative" food and whiteness (e.g., Alkon & McCullen 2011), and the added surveillance and institutional racism encountered by mothers of color (Elliott et al. 2016).

While women from a range of race and class positions engage in calibration to achieve distance from both the McDonald's Mom and the Organic Mom, they do not engage with them on an even playing field. Both the social threat associated with these maternal figures, and the flexibility mothers experience in their calibration efforts, are deeply shaped by their ethno-racial and classed positions. First, while both figures are stigmatized, they bring uneven penalties. Within the context of neoliberal healthism and the moral panic of the "obesity epidemic", the stigma of being perceived as an inattentive, "bad" feeder is likely to be much more socially shameful, and thus to engender significantly more discrimination and surveillance than the overachieving feeder, who is seen as uptight, controlling, or elitist (Boero 2010; Elliot et al. 2016; Wright, Maher & Tanner 2015). Because lower class mothers are more discursively tied to the McDonald's Mom, they are more likely to be labeled and suffer the disproportionately negative effects than others. Second, class positioning shapes the economic and cultural capital available to mothers as they navigate these stigmatized figures. In particular, the challenge of feeding children on a limited income makes calibrating the standards of idealized maternal foodwork difficult. In other words, class shapes the relative proximity of mothers to each of these figures, and thus the degree of distancing required of them through calibration, as well as the resources they have available to them in the calibration process. Our findings nonetheless indicate that women across classes perform this calibration work, suggesting the resonance of these figures in contemporary discourses of maternal feeding.

Given the relational constitution of mother and child, our analysis also offers insight into contemporary childhood ideals. While the McDonald's Mom and the Organic Mom may appear as polar opposites, we find a striking point of similarity in their construction: namely, both pathologized maternal figures fail to produce a child who exercises good choices. The McDonald's Mom encourages *bad* choices by providing children with a diet of fast foods and processed snacks. By contrast, the Organic Mom's overbearing feeding strategies leave her children with no capacity to exercise choices on their own, thus similarly failing to socialize them to be responsible eaters. In both cases, the stigmatized maternal figure produces an improperly socialized child, and a central component of that failure is the production of a consumer who is unable to make informed choices – a hallmark of consumer citizenship in a neoliberal era (Cairns & Johnston 2015b; Guthman 2008). By contrast, the idealized "good mother" is constructed in relation to the well-socialized child-eater who can visit McDonald's once a year and choose to eat a diversity of vegetables, thereby embodying the next generation of neoliberal consumer-citizens assuming individual responsibility for their health and well-being.

References

Alkon, A.H. & McCullen, C.G., 2011, 'Whiteness and farmers markets: Performances, perpetuations ... contestations?', *Antipode*, vol. 43, no. 4, pp. 937–959.

Beagan, B., Chapman, G.E., D'Sylva, A., & Bassett, B.R., 2008, '"It's just easier for me to do it": Rationalizing the family division of food-work', *Sociology*, vol. 42, no. 4, pp. 653–671.

Beagan, B., Chapman, G.E., Johnston, J., McPhail, D., Powers, E. & Valliantos, H., 2014, *Acquired Tastes: Why Families Eat the Way they Do*, UBC Press, Vancouver.

Bianchi, S.M., Milkie, M.A., Sayer, L.C., & Robinson, J.P., 2000, 'Is anyone doing the housework? Trends in the gender division of household labor', *Social forces*, vol. 79, no. 1, pp. 191–228.

Boero, N., 2010, 'Fat kids, working moms, and the epidemic of obesity: Race, class, and mother-blame', in E. Rothblum & S. Solovay (eds.), *The Fat Studies Reader*, New York University Press, New York, pp. 113–119.

Bowen, S., Elliott, S., & Brenton, J., 2014, 'The joy of cooking?', *Contexts*, vol. 13, no. 3, pp. 20–25.

Bugge, A.B. & Almas, R., 2006, 'Domestic dinner: Representations and practices of a proper meal among young suburban mothers', *Journal of Consumer Culture*, vol. 6, pp. 203–228.

Burman, E. & Stacey, J., 2010, 'The child and childhood in feminist theory', *Feminist Theory*, vol. 11, no. 3, pp. 224–227.

Cairns, K., DeLaat, K., Johnston, J., & Baumann, S., 2014, 'The caring, committed eco-mom', in B. Barendregt & R. Jaffe (eds.), *Green Consumption: The Global Rise of Eco-Chic*, Bloomsbury Publishing, London, pp. 100–114.

Cairns, K. & Johnston, J., 2015a, *Food and Femininity*, Bloomsbury, London.

Cairns, K. & Johnston, J., 2015b, 'Choosing health: Embodied neoliberalism, post-feminism, and the "do-diet"', *Theory and Society*, vol. 44, pp. 153–175.

Cairns, K., Johnston, J. & MacKendrick, N., 2013, 'Feeding the "organic child": Mothering through ethical consumption', *Journal of Consumer Culture*, vol. 13, no. 2, pp. 97–118.

Charles, N. & Kerr, M., 1988, *Women, Food and Families*, Manchester University Press, Manchester, UK.

Chesler, P., 1974, *Women and Madness*, Avon Books, New York.

Cook, D., 2009, 'Semantic provisioning of children's food: Commerce, care and maternal practice', *Childhood*, vol. 16, no. 3, pp. 317–334.

Daniel, C., 2016, 'Economic constraints on taste formation and the true cost of healthy eating', *Social Science & Medicine*, vol. 148, pp. 34–41.

DeVault, M., 1991, *Feeding the Family: The Social Organization of Caring as Gendered Work*, University of Chicago Press, Chicago.

Elliott, S., Bowen, S., Brenton, J., Hardison-Moody, A., 2016, 'Intersectionality and food justice: Lessons from a community-based, participatory project about maternal food-work', Paper presented at Scarborough Fare: Global Foodways and Local Foods in a Transnational City, the annual meetings of the Association for the Study of Food and Society, June 15–22, Toronto, ON, University of Toronto.

Goffman, E., 1963, *Stigma: Notes on the Management of Spoiled Identity*, Prentice Hall, Englewood Cliffs, NJ.

Guthman, J., 2008, 'Neoliberalism and the making of food politics in California', *Geoforum*, vol. 39, no. 3, pp. 1171–1183.

Hays, S., 1996, *The Cultural Contradictions of Motherhood*, Yale University Press, New Haven.

Herndon, A.M., 2010, 'Mommy made me do it: Mothering fat children in the midst of the obesity epidemic', *Food, Culture & Society*, vol. 13, no. 3, pp. 331–349.

Johnston, J. & BaumannS., 2015 [2010], *Foodies: Democracy and Distinction in the Gourmet Foodscape*, Routledge, New York.

Ladd-Taylor, M. & Umansky, L., 1998, 'Introduction', in M. Ladd-Taylor & L. Umansky (eds.), *Bad Mothers: The Politics of Blame in Twentieth-Century America*, New York University Press, New York, pp. 1–28.

Link, B.G. & Phelan, J.C., 2001, 'Conceptualizing stigma', *Annual Review of Sociology*, vol. 27, no. 1, pp. 363–385.

Lupton, D., 1996, *Food, the Body and the Self*, Sage, London.

Lupton, D., 2014, 'Precious, pure, uncivilized, vulnerable: Infant embodiment in Australian popular media', *Children & Society*, vol. 28, pp. 341–351.

Mackendrick, N., 2014, 'More work for mother: Chemical body burdens as a maternal responsibility', *Gender & Society*, vol. 28, no. 5, pp. 705–728.

MacKendrick, N. & Stevens, L.M., 2016, '"Taking back a little bit of control": Managing the contaminated body through consumption', *Sociological Forum*, vol. 31, no. 2, pp. 310–329.

MacKendrick, N. & Pristavec, T., 2016, 'Between careful and crazy: Foodwork as a balancing act', Paper presented at Scarborough Fare: Global Foodways and Local Foods in a Transnational City, the annual meetings of the Association for the Study of Food and Society, June 15–22, Toronto, Ontario, University of Toronto.

Malson, H., 1998, *The Thin Woman: Feminism, Post-Structuralism and Anorexia Nervosa*, Routledge, New York.

Murphy, E., 2000, 'Risk, responsibility, and rhetoric in infant feeding', *Journal of Contemporary Ethnography*, vol. 29, no. 3, pp. 291–325.

O'Connell, R. & Brannen, J., 2016, *Food, Families and Work*, Bloomsbury, New York.

Paddock, J., 2015, 'Positioning food cultures: "Alternative" food as distinctive consumer practice', *Sociology*, pp. 1–17, Doi: doi:10.1177/0038038515585474.

Sayer, L.C., 2005, 'Gender, time and inequality: Trends in women's and men's paid work, unpaid work and free time', *Social forces*, vol. 84, no. 1, pp. 285–303.

Szabo, M., 2014, 'Men nurturing through food: Challenging gender dichotomies around domestic cooking', *Journal of Gender Studies*, vol. 23, no. 1, pp. 18–31.

Warin, M., Zivkovic, T., Moore, V. & Davies, M., 2012, 'Mothers as smoking guns: Fetal overnutrition and the reproduction of obesity', *Feminism & Psychology*, vol. 22, no. 3, pp. 360–375.

Wright, J., Maher, J. & Tanner, C., 2015, 'Social class, anxieties and mothers' foodwork', *Sociology of health & illness*, vol. 37, no. 3, pp. 422–436.

Chapter 12

When intensive mothering becomes a necessity

Feeding children on the ketogenic diet

Michelle Webster

The ketogenic diet

The ketogenic diet is a high fat, low carbohydrate diet that has traditionally been used to treat drug-resistant childhood epilepsy (Farasat et al., 2006). It was originally introduced as a treatment for epilepsy in 1921, but its use declined with the introduction of a new antiepileptic drug in 1938 (Hartman and Vining, 2007; Wheless, 2008). However, over the past 15–20 years there has been a resurgence of interest in the diet in both the United States and the UK (Wheless, 2008; Payne et al., 2011).

Although the exact mechanisms of the diet are still unknown (Neal et al., 2008), it controls seizures by mimicking the metabolic effects of starvation (Payne et al., 2011; Cross, 2012). This is achieved through the diet being high in fat and low in carbohydrate in order to produce ketosis (a metabolic state where the body uses ketones rather than glucose for energy) (Payne et al., 2011). Alternatives to the ketogenic diet have also been introduced; they include the Medium Chain Triglyceride (MCT) ketogenic diet and the Modified Atkins Diet (MAD) (Payne et al., 2011). Both are intended to improve palatability by increasing the flexibility of the diet and by allowing higher amounts of protein and carbohydrate (Payne et al., 2011). Although the MAD is not medically defined as a 'ketogenic diet', for the purposes of this chapter it will be referred to as such due to its high fat content.

The ratio of fat to protein and carbohydrate on the ketogenic diet varies between 2:1 and 4:1, meaning patients receive up to 80% of their calories in the form of fat (Cross, 2012; Ferrie et al., 2012c). The MAD and classical diets rely on large amounts of butter, cream and mayonnaise for their high fat content (Ferrie et al., 2012c) while the MCT diet uses MCT oil and Liquigen. Other than the type of fat that each diet uses, the main difference between the diets is that protein is not limited on the MAD.

The majority of research into the ketogenic diet thus far has been from a biological perspective and little has been written regarding use of the diet on a daily basis in the home. One exception is a recent paper by Webster and Gabe (2016), which explores the meanings parents attached to foods when using the ketogenic diet. This chapter will extend our understanding of how this diet is incorporated into family life by exploring the extent of the food work that went into implementing the diet, who took responsibility for this food work and how food work impacted on mothering identity.

Mothering and food work

Within sociological theory it is argued that we are living in a 'risk society' (Beck, 1992) where risk consciousness is high, i.e. individuals use the notion of risk to organise their social worlds (Giddens, 1991). With risk consciousness now more pervasive, social actors have become increasingly 'individualised' (Beck, 1992; Beck and Beck-Gernsheim, 2002). Beck argues that in the past individuals were restricted by social structures and customs, whereas they are now more reflexive, have greater freedom over the choices they can make and, consequently, biographies are 'self-produced' (Beck, 1992: 135). However, Beck and Beck-Gernsheim (2002) note that individualisation is a double-edged sword, as although people now have more freedom, they are also deemed to be responsible for the choices they make. Moreover, with children being conceptualised as a particularly 'at risk' group (Jackson and Scott, 1999; Lupton, 1999; Firkins and Candlin, 2006; Meyer, 2007; Lee et al., 2010), individualisation has resulted in parents being seen as responsible for protecting their children from risks (Jackson and Scott, 1999; Geinger et al., 2013). Indeed, 'what arises from it [the construction of the child "at risk"] is the construction of the parent as a *manager of risks*' (Lee et al., 2014: 12 original emphasis).

One way in which parents try to manage risks is through what has been termed 'intensive parenting' (see Cairns *et al.*, this volume). Hoffman argues this type of parenting is where parents 'micromanage all aspects of their children's lives in an effort to protect the child from adverse experiences' (2010: 387). Hoffman (2010) also believes this style of parenting is a direct reaction to a climate of risk. It has been argued that intensive parenting practices are largely gender specific, with predominantly mothers adjusting their family practices in accordance with this ideology (Hays, 1996; Vincent and Ball, 2007; Shirani et al., 2012). Furthermore, intensive parenting has also been found to be class specific (Vincent and Ball, 2007). Vincent and Ball argue that intensive parenting specifically applies to the middle classes who view their children as 'a project – soft, malleable and able to be developed and improved' (2007: 1066). Working class parents, on the other hand, were found to believe that their children would develop appropriately as long as they provided love, food and safety (Vincent and Ball, 2007).

Hays (1996) argues that although intensive mothering ideology may not be followed in practice by every mother, there is still the assumption that intensive mothering constitutes 'proper' mothering. Intensive mothering ideology has permeated all aspects of mothering practice and food work is no exception. For instance, although women spend less time cooking in contemporary society, Dixon and Banwell (2004) found that the women in their study spent the same amount of time worrying about the meals they were going to prepare. Harman and Cappellini (2015) have also illustrated the amount of work that mothers put into preparing their children's lunchboxes in order to please a variety of audiences, including their child and the child's school.

Despite intensive mothering practices feeding into women's food practices, food work as a form of women's work is by no means a new phenomenon. Similar to other forms of domestic labour, it has been found that women take on the majority of the cooking work within the family (Calnan and Williams, 1991; Dixon and Banwell, 2004; Curtis et al., 2009; Metcalfe et al., 2009). Furthermore, feeding the family has particular significance for women's identities as love and care are displayed through this practice (DeVault 1991; Lupton, 1996; Kaplan, 2000; Devine et al., 2003; Cook, 2009b; Curtis et al., 2009; James et al., 2009; Metcalfe et al., 2009). Indeed, Dixon and Banwell (2004) found that mothers spent a considerable amount of time planning meals because they felt that satisfying the desires of their family members was an important part of their lives.

In addition to food work, care work is another form of labour that has traditionally been seen as women's work. Indeed, it is widely acknowledged that women continue to provide the bulk of informal care within the family (Davis and Greenstein, 2004; McKie et al., 2004; Chambers, 2012). Use of the ketogenic diet, and dietary treatment more generally within the family, is an interesting area to explore as the work that goes into implementing the diet is simultaneously food work and care work. Given the existing literature, it would be reasonable to assume that the majority of this work is undertaken by women. This chapter explores whether this is the case, the extent of the work that goes into implementing the ketogenic diet on a daily basis and how this work can impact on parenting identity. But first, the methodology used to collect the data that this chapter draws on is outlined and discussed below.

Methodology

The data presented within this chapter are drawn from a broader study focusing on the experience and management of childhood epilepsy within the family. A qualitative approach was taken in order to explore parents' experiences of using the ketogenic diet to treat their children's epilepsy. The research was advertised through three UK based charities: *Epilepsy Action*, *The Daisy Garland* and *Matthew's Friends*. The charities placed adverts on their websites, online forums, social media pages, and in their newsletters.

In-depth semi-structured interviews were carried out with 12 parents from 10 families. All families were two-parent families and had between two and four children. The children on the diet consisted of four girls and six boys aged between three and 10 years. Seven of the children were on the classical version of the diet, two were on the MCT diet and one was on the MAD. Overall, the data presented below comprise the views of 10 mothers and two fathers (where both parents from one family participated they were interviewed together). The great majority of participants were White British or White European, with one parent being Asian (foreign-born). Although the families were from a range of socioeconomic groups, the majority were in the top quartile of earners.

Six interviews were conducted face-to-face, two were phone interviews, one was conducted via Skype and one was an email interview. It was not possible to conduct all of the interviews face-to-face due to the location of some of the participants; those who were interviewed face-to-face were all from mainland UK, those who were interviewed over the phone were from non-mainland UK and the Skype and email interviews were with parents from Western Europe and Eastern Europe (all the interviews were conducted in English).

The interviews lasted between one and two hours and focused on the child's food consumption and parents' daily routine in relation to implementing the diet. Parents often gave very rich answers and used stories to illustrate their points. Consequently, parents also brought up: their child's food preferences, preparation time, cost, managing the diet on special occasions, difficulties associated with implementing the diet, how they fitted the diet into their daily lives and others' reactions to the diet. If the participants themselves did not raise these topics they were probed about them.

All interviews were audio-recorded and transcribed *verbatim*, with the exception of the email interview. The data were then coded using NVivo 10 and analysed using a constructivist grounded theory approach (Charmaz, 2006). In contrast to Glaser and Strauss' (1999) grounded theory, a literature review was conducted prior to carrying out the interviews in order to gain an understanding of previous research on similar topics. But, in accordance with Glaser and Strauss (1999), themes were developed using the constant comparative method throughout the data collection phase, emerging themes were drawn upon in later interviews to fill gaps in the analysis, and participants were recruited until categories became saturated.

Ethical approval was granted by the Centre for Criminology and Sociology's departmental ethics committee at Royal Holloway, University of London prior to beginning data collection. In line with this approval, participants and their family members are referred to using pseudonyms to maintain their anonymity.

Below, the findings from the study are reported. To begin, the extent of the food work that went into implementing the diet will be explained. Following on from this, the gendered nature of this food work will be outlined. Finally, the expert carer role will be introduced and the way in which mothering identity was affected by the mental, emotional and physical labour that constituted intensive mothering will be explored.

The necessity of intensive parenting

Within this section the extent of the food work that surrounded children's food consumption will be illustrated. It is argued that the care, attention and effort that went into planning, preparing and monitoring children's food consumption can be described as intensive parenting (see Boni, this volume). Furthermore, this type of parenting was necessary within these families in order to ensure that the child's treatment was administered correctly and adhered to on a daily basis.

All children on the ketogenic diet had a prescription for their food consumption that specified the amount of fat, protein and carbohydrate that each of their meals, and the entirety of their food consumption, had to contain. The intensive aspect of parenting that these prescriptions necessitated was that parents had to spend a considerable amount of time working out meal plans that not only adhered to the child's prescription, but importantly, that their child would want to eat. Parents did receive support from dieticians and when they had planned menus they could repeat them, but if they wanted to change any of the ingredients, or even change the brand of a product they were using, they would need to recalculate the meal to ensure it was of the correct nutritional value. One mother went further and explained that she even checked the fat content on cream because it varied at different times of year. Furthermore, like most children, the children on the diet sometimes went through phases and they would go off foods that they had previously enjoyed. For instance, Rachel explained:

> She gets fed up with the same thing everyday and so you've always got to be one step ahead, thinking "right she's going to go off this soon". You can see when she starts to like fiddle with her food that she's going off it. So I've always got to be thinking "right, what can I give her next?"

Consequently, parents were often trying to think of new recipes to make sure that their children would eat the food that they had prepared and so their children were enjoying what they were eating. Thinking of new recipes often resulted in additional time and effort because it sometimes required a process of trial and error; parents would occasionally plan a meal that worked on paper, but when they cooked it they felt the final product was not edible. Similarly, children did not always like the new meals that their parents created and when this happened the challenge of needing to design new menus would start again.

A further way in which planning children's food consumption was intensified was that planning shopping lists and days out also needed additional consideration. Parents had to ensure that they had purchased everything they needed for their child's meals, as if they ran out of a particular product it was not always easy to find an alternative from stock cupboard items. Furthermore, on days out parents often needed to prepare food to take with them (making sure food items would travel and stay fresh, particularly during the summer). Hannah, for example, said:

> We have a couple of places that we can go to that are happy that we bring our food with us for Jack. I just do his lunch; his chicken, beans and butter in a flask … and the hotel put it onto the plate for me. So it came out at the same time as everybody else's, so he feels part of it.

Like Hannah suggests above, some restaurants and cafes would accommodate families and let them bring their own foods, whereas others were not happy for this to happen. Some parents would instead research different restaurants' menus and plan where may be a suitable place to eat; this often meant parents would take scales with them to measure their child's portion.

Another way in which parenting surrounding children's food consumption comprised intensive parenting was that the children's foods had to be accurately measured. In order to ensure that children were receiving their correct prescription each ingredient had to be weighed to the gram. One parent went even further, as Naomi is explaining below:

> Actually I probably weigh things a lot more accurately than some people would because, you know, I have 5.6 grams of something. Whereas I think the dietician probably thinks I'm a bit over the top with that but I know exactly that she's getting the right ratio every single time.

Here Naomi is explaining that she weighed her daughter's food down to one decimal place and that this enabled her to feel confident that she was treating her daughter's condition as best she could. Although Naomi was the only parent to weigh her child's food to one decimal place, the accuracy that the parents talked about was a significant aspect of their explanations of food preparation.

As well as the planning and preparation of children's food on the ketogenic diet amounting to intensive parenting, parents also closely monitored their children when they were around food; this was partly to ensure that children consumed all of their food (to make sure they got their full prescription) and also to make certain that they did not consume any foods outside of their prescription. For instance, if a child was to eat some sweets or a piece of chocolate, this would bring them out of ketosis and undermine the therapeutic value of the diet. Jane illustrated this when she recalled a recent incident:

> His head teacher handed him a piece of bread in church the other day and didn't think. Luckily enough myself and my husband were there, and Toby's the type of child who wouldn't cheat on it, but if you had a child that would then, you know, I think it would be a lot harder.

Jane's extract demonstrates the constant vigilance that parents felt was necessary in order to successfully implement the diet. Food features in many aspects of daily life and is often used as a treat for children; parents became acutely aware of this when their children were on the ketogenic diet. Furthermore, as Jane's quote suggests, parents also had to spend time informing others about their child's diet and the need to monitor their food consumption, particularly those who, at times, took responsibility for caring for the child. Indeed, one of the most frustrating experiences for parents was when other people did not understand how it important it was for their child to adhere to the diet after it had been explained to them. A few parents felt that occasionally others saw them as neurotic parents who had put their child on a fad diet.

Within this section the intensive nature of planning and preparing foods on the ketogenic diet as well as monitoring children's food consumption has been outlined. It is argued that due to the nature of the ketogenic diet, this treatment requires this intensive approach to parenting. Thus far, it has been suggested that the ketogenic diet necessitated intensive *parenting*, however, what this translated to in many families was in fact intensive *mothering*, which is discussed in the following section.

The gendered nature of food work

All of the 10 families that took part in the research were two parent families and the fathers in all of these families worked full-time. Three of the mothers also worked full-time, four worked part-time and three described themselves as a carer (for their child with epilepsy) and/or a homemaker. Although many of the mothers that took part in the study were in employment as well as the father, the majority of the food work required to implement the diet was carried out by the mothers; consequently, it was intensive mothering that was enacted in the majority of these families.

In only two of the families did the father prepare any of the child's meals and Ana explained 'we cannot have a day off, which more or less was sometimes the subject of an argument between me and my husband – who will prepare the meal for Stefan'. Ana's quote illustrates that the work that went into implementing the diet was required seven days a week for the duration that the child was on the diet. Furthermore, mothers always contributed to the food work relating to the diet, whereas only a minority of fathers did. Indeed, when Rachel was asked if she prepared all her daughter's meals she said:

It is just me. My husband wouldn't have a clue. If she ever goes to stay at my Mum's or my mother-in-law's I have to like weigh everything out beforehand and put them in different lunchboxes, give them instructions on how to cook it. My husband will feed her. Because we have to feed her because we have to make sure she gets all the oil, all the mayonnaise, because otherwise she would just pick the nice bits off the plate and leave it all. So my husband's quite good at doing that. But then he doesn't get home from work until about 7 o'clock at night so I'm pretty much doing it all by myself anyway, which is a strain. It is hard. But I'm getting used to it now.

This extract shows that even when others were feeding the child the mother often still had to do the majority of the food preparation. Similarly to Rachel's description, in families where someone fed the child, fathers would sometimes share this responsibility with their partner. Although Rachel mentions her husband's work schedule as a reason for his inability to do more during the week, in one family where both parents worked full-time the mother still prepared all her child's meals.

In two other families, fathers contributed to the implementation of the diet in other ways; for instance, one father created new recipes using the EKM (Electronic Ketogenic Manager – a computer package that can be used to create meal plans adhering to the child's prescription) and another would crush his son's tablets daily because the child could not swallow tablets and the syrup version of the same drug contained sugar that he was not allowed on the diet. Although these fathers were caring for their children, the tasks they undertook were somewhat peripheral to the bulk of the time consuming labour that mothers took on. Furthermore, in two of the families mothers cited their daughters as being more helpful than their husbands in terms of thinking of new recipes and helping with food preparation (Webster, 2018).

In the majority of the families the fathers did not contribute to any food preparation within the family more generally. However, in one family where both parents worked full-time the father did prepare meals for other family members during the week, but not the child on the diet. It is suggested that, in accordance with traditional gender roles, it was not only because the diet was food work, but also because it was care work, that meant women undertook the majority of the work in these families.

Looking at the 10 families as a whole, it was mothers who contributed the vast majority of the physical labour, such as shopping, food preparation and feeding children. Mothers also provided the best part of the mental labour of deciding what the child would eat, what needed to be purchased and communicating with others to ensure that those caring for the child were fully informed about the diet. Additionally, it was overwhelmingly mothers who supplied the emotional labour of ensuring children felt loved and included in social situations surrounding food. For example, they would create ketogenic alternatives of foods to fulfil children's requests for particular foods and so that children could eat foods that were similar to those that others were eating (Webster and Gabe, 2016).

All the families that took part in this study had success on the ketogenic diet and felt that their children had benefitted from this treatment. The hard work that mothers put into implementing the diet was rewarded because they could see the positive results of their efforts and many saw the diet as a saviour, which is discussed below.

Treatment as a saviour

A common theme in mothers' discussions was that they felt guilty when they initially started treating their child's epilepsy with the ketogenic diet. For instance, Jane explained 'you feel guilty because you're taking so much away from them'. Upon initiating the diet parents had to deny their children foods that they requested and that they had previously enjoyed because they were not allowed on the diet. This was one of the aspects of this particular dietary treatment that parents found emotionally troubling. However, when the diet proved to be successful this helped them to overcome these feelings of guilt as they felt the benefit that the treatment was having was worthwhile.

For 6 of the 10 families using the diet, a reduction in seizures and emergency hospital admissions meant that the ketogenic diet was seen in a literal sense as a lifesaver. For instance, Naomi said:

> We have seen a significant improvement. In fact, September this year we will have been two years out of hospital ... Unfortunately we're not one of the small few for who it completely stops the seizures, but it's given me back my daughter without a doubt.

For Naomi, and others in a similar situation, success on the ketogenic diet meant that they had gone from regular emergency admissions to hospital to few or none. This treatment, therefore, was not only a saviour of the child's life but also for the family as a whole who no longer, or very rarely, had to go through the process of seeing their child or sibling admitted to hospital. The diet, consequently, provided a form of much valued stability for these families.

In Naomi's extract above she talks about getting her daughter 'back'. This same feeling was expressed by a further three parents. Some felt regaining their child was a result of a reduction in drug treatment, whereas others felt it was attributable to the diet itself, as Hannah explained:

> The diet hasn't given us seizure freedom or much control really. The drugs are still controlling it to a certain extent. But the diet has given us

Jack's personality. Jack is much clearer in his thinking and himself. It's like we've got his little personality back.

For these families the diet was again seen as a saviour, as they felt they had regained the child's personality, which was previously seen to be lost.

Two additional mothers, however, did not feel they had regained their child, but rather that they had seen them for the first time. For instance, Hashani said 'it's like somebody reached in and switched her on'. Similarly, Kelly commented 'it's like having a child that was running on 10% now running on like 80, 85%'. Therefore, like the mothers above, Hashani and Kelly felt that they had been able to access elements of their children's personalities that had previously been lost. All the mothers who expressed sentiments of regaining their child or seeing their personality for the first time also spoke about what this meant for the child; they all felt that their children were happier as they were more able to participate in activities because they experienced fewer debilitating side effects from the condition and/or drug treatments.

Because mothers held such overwhelming positive views of the diet it meant that they could feel that their hard work had paid off as they were able to improve their child's quality of life, and often the quality of life of other family members as a result. Following on from mothers' views of the diet as a saviour, it will be argued that the parents implementing this diet, and mothers in particular, had become expert carers, which is the focus of the following section.

Expert carers

Within medical sociology considerable attention has been given to lay expertise (Prior, 2003). It is argued that those with chronic conditions build up a detailed knowledge of their conditions and their bodies (Whelan, 2007; Busby et al., 1997). Here, this notion is extended to argue that the mothers that took part in this study had become expert carers; this enabled them to overcome the feelings of guilt, mentioned above, and feel they were being good mothers. Indeed, these mothers were experts in a number of different ways.

Firstly, mothers were experts at implementing the diet. As was described above, they were experts at measuring food, calculating new recipes that fulfilled their child's prescription and they were experts at monitoring their children to ensure that they adhered to the diet. Secondly, mothers were experts on their own children. They possessed a detailed knowledge of their children's mannerisms and their food likes and dislikes. Indeed, as Harman and Cappellini (2015) illustrate in their work on lunchboxes, mothers' in-depth understanding of their children's food preferences enabled them to personalise lunchboxes to fulfil the children's desires. In this instance, as a result of this knowledge, mothers could create recipes for their children that they thought they would like. They could also detect when their children were starting to go off particular meals, which enabled them to have alternatives lined up ready. Furthermore, in consultation with the dieticians, the mothers were able to select the diet that they thought would be most suitable for their child from the beginning. For instance, Kelly described her reasoning for selecting the MCT diet for her son:

> They [dieticians] explained to me about the three diets. And Ryan ... as he's got a bit older he enjoys food. So I didn't want to take that away from him and I wanted to keep him eating things that he enjoyed eating, even if it was less. Because when children have Dravet [a particular epilepsy syndrome] they can sometimes have poor muscle tone and Ryan does have that so he's never been good at eating meat. You know, because it requires a lot of chewing. So we thought the classical one, if he was required to eat a lot of meat and things like that, it just wouldn't be sustainable. And the Atkins diet, that modified Atkins one as well, we thought it was too much in the way of meat on that. So that's why I went for the MCT one.

Although families did sometimes change diets, mothers' knowledge of their children informed decisions regarding which diet was most suitable for their child, as Kelly's extract illustrates. In this sense, mothers were expert carers because their relationships with their children helped them to select the most appropriate diet and to continue implementing the diet on a daily basis whilst keeping their children as happy with their food consumption as possible.

Lastly, by being experts at implementing the diet and experts on their children, this meant that mothers were also experts at treating their child's condition. This aspect of the expert carer role was extremely important for mothering identity as it enabled mothers to overcome the feelings of guilt that were provoked by having to deny their children certain foods.

Interestingly, many of the mothers described how they had initially been told that the ketogenic diet was not a viable option for their child and that they had had to push to be allowed to try this treatment. Jessica, for example, said 'we pleaded for it'. The children in these families had all tried a number of medications that had not successfully controlled their seizures and many had experienced side effects as a result of drug treatment. Similarly to Jessica, Naomi explained how she:

> Had to battle for it. Because initially when I spoke to our local consultant about it he had quite negative ideas about the diet I think, and told us it was unpalatable and it would be too hard to do and she was too young and all this sort of stuff. But the drugs weren't working and

we were in hospital almost weekly and her development was most definitely stagnating and she was losing acquired skills as well. So it did feel very much, a last resort I suppose. I wasn't willing to try any more different drugs. I knew there was quite a few still we could try but once they've failed two, the chances of another drug working is very small. And obviously you've got all the nasty side effects and everything so, yeah, so I was quite passionate that I wanted to try the diet.

As these families had all had negative experiences with previous drug treatments and they had all had success on the diet, mothers could feel that their efforts had been worthwhile and that they had done what was right for their child. Indeed, as was outlined above, many of these parents saw the diet as a saviour. As a result, these mothers could feel like expert carers as they had made decisions that had directly benefitted their child's health when medical professionals had sometimes discouraged such efforts.

It is undeniable that mothers found the intensive physical, mental and emotional labour that went into implementing the diet challenging and/or draining at times. However, the sacrifices they were making also helped them to feel they were being good mothers. Indeed, always putting the child first is a central aspect of intensive mothering (Hays, 1996). Furthermore, through being expert carers mothers could take credit for their hard work and the positive impact their efforts had on their child's health.

Discussion

The intensive mothering ideology is often critiqued as it results in additional pressure being placed on women in order for them to be viewed by themselves and others as good mothers (Hays, 1996). However, this chapter has illustrated that in some instances intensive parenting is a necessity. It was necessary for parents to spend additional time on and pay close attention to the planning, preparation and consumption of their children's food; for instance, all meals had to be planned and foods had to be weighed. This intensive parenting was required so that children's meals fulfilled their prescriptions and so that children were happy to adhere to dietary restrictions.

On the other hand, although it can be argued that intensive parenting was a necessity, intensive mothering was not. Despite this, it was mothers that took on the majority of the work that went into implementing the diet. Although food work is not equally distributed between males and females more generally (Calnan and Williams, 1991; Dixon and Banwell, 2004; Curtis et al., 2009; Metcalfe et al., 2009), it is argued here that because dietary treatment is a combination of food work and care work, both of which are predominantly undertaken by women, mothers in these families contributed more to the implementation of this treatment than their partners. Indeed, even when fathers contributed to some of the food preparation or feeding tasks, it was mothers that undertook the majority of the mental and emotional labour that made the diet a success on a daily basis (see Gram and Grønhøj, this volume).

Furthermore, the concept of the expert carer has been introduced in this chapter. Previous discussions on lay experts (Whelan, 2007; Busby et al., 1997) have been extended here, as it has been shown that it is not only the person with the chronic condition that can become an 'expert'. It has been argued that these mothers were expert carers for three main reasons. Firstly, they were experts at implementing the diet – they were able to measure all their child's food so that the child's food consumption fulfilled their prescription and mothers were also able to create new recipes whilst adhering to dietary restrictions. Secondly, mothers were experts on their children; this enabled them to construct meals that their children enjoyed, which again meant that the diet was implemented successfully. Thirdly, the expertise already discussed meant that mothers were experts at treating their child's condition; this was particularly significant as previous treatments had not been successful and mothers often reported that they had to work hard to convince medical professionals to allow them to try the ketogenic diet. Additionally, it was shown that mothers talked about this diet as a saviour. All the families that took part in this study had had success on the diet and seeing treatment in this way again meant that mothers' could feel that they were being good mothers as they were putting their child first. Furthermore, the sacrifices mothers were making in terms of the physical, mental and emotional labour that went into implementing the diet had resulted in improvements in the child's health and wellbeing. Consequently, it is argued that intensive mothering practices and the development of caring expertise directly impacted on mothering identity, as this helped mothers to overcome some of the negative emotions associated with denying children certain foods.

Families using the ketogenic diet are strongly encouraged to trial the diet for three months in order to determine whether it will be an effective treatment for the child. It is clear that mothers' views on the efficacy of diet impacted on the way they felt about the work they put into implementing it on a daily basis. Future research could explore the views of parents, and mothers in particular, who have undertaken these intensive mothering practices surrounding food and found that the diet was not effective. There is the potential that their efforts may still contribute to a good mother identity because they made sacrifices for their child. Alternatively, they may feel they have failed. Furthermore, it would be of interest to know how mothering identity is affected in families who decide to discontinue the diet prior to the three-month mark.

Overall, this chapter has demonstrated that the care work and food work that went into implementing the ketogenic diet were heavily gendered with mothers taking on the majority of the responsibility. As a result, it has also been shown that mothers can develop expertise on treating their child's chronic condition and that the expert carer roles makes them feel that their efforts are worthwhile and that they are being good mothers. Furthermore, it has been argued that intensive parenting is not always a result of cultural ideology, as there are some situations that require intensive parenting practices. It was, however, in part this ideology that resulted in positive implications for mothering identity. Therefore, these mothers' experiences were not only influenced by the efficacy of the diet, but also by societal norms.

References

Beck, U. (1992) *Risk Society: Towards a New Modernity*, London: Sage.
Beck, U. & Beck-Gernsheim, E. (2002) *Individualization: Institutionalized Individualism and its Social and Political Consequences*, London: Sage.
Busby, H., Williams, G. & Rogers, A. (1997) 'Bodies of knowledge: Lay and biomedical understandings of musculoskeletal disease', *Sociology of Health and Illness*, 19(19B):79–99.
Calnan, M. & Williams, S. (1991) 'Style of life and the salience of health: An exploratory study of health related practices in households from differing socio-economic circumstances', *Sociology of Health and Illness*, 13(4):506–529.
Chambers, D. (2012) *A sociology of Family Life: Change and Diversity in Intimate Relationships*, Cambridge: Polity Press.
Davis, S. & Greenstein, T. (2004) 'Cross-national variations in the division of household labor', *Journal of Marriage and Family*, 66(5):1260–1271.
Cook, D. (2009) 'Children's subjectivities and commercial meaning: The delicate battle mothers wage when feeding their children', in A. James, A. Kjorholt & V. Tingstad [Eds] *Children, Food and Identity in Everyday Life*, Basingstoke: Palgrave Macmillan, pp. 112–129.
Cross, J.H. (2012) 'Ketogenic diet in the management of childhood epilepsy', in G. Alarcón & A. Valentín [Eds] *Introduction to Epilepsy*, Cambridge: Cambridge University Press, pp. 456–457.
Curtis, P., James, A. & Ellis, K. (2009) 'Fathering through food: Children's perceptions of fathers' contributions to family food practices', in A. James, A. Kjorholt & V. Tingstad [Eds] *Children, Food and Identity in Everyday Life*, Basingstoke: Palgrave Macmillan, pp. 94–111.
DeVault, M.L. (1991) *Feeding the Family: The Social Organization of Caring as Gendered Work*, London: The University of Chicago Press.
Devine, C., Connors, M.M., Sobal, J. & Bisogni, C.A. (2003) 'Sandwiching it in: Spillover of work onto food choices and family roles in low- and moderate-income urban households', *Social Sciences and Medicine*, 56(3):617–630.
Dixon, J. & Banwell, C. (2004) 'Heading the table: Parenting and the junior consumer', *British Food Journal*, 106(2/3):181–193.
Farasat, S., Kossoff, E.H., Pillas, D.J., Rubenstein, J.E., Vining, E.P. & Freeman, J.E. (2006) 'The importance of parental expectations of cognitive improvement for their children with epilepsy prior to starting the ketogenic diet', *Epilepsy and Behavior*, 8:406–410.

Ferrie, C.D., Smithson, W.H. & Walker, M.C. (2012) 'Non-drug treatments including epilepsy surgery', in W.H. Smithson & M.C. Walker [Eds] *ABC of Epilepsy*, Chichester: Wiley-Blackwell, pp. 18–20.

Firkins, A. & Candlin, C.N. (2006) 'Framing the child at risk', *Health, Risk and Society*, 8(3): 273–291.

Geinger, F., Vandenbroeck, M. & Roets, G. (2013) 'Parenting as performance: Parents as consumers and (de)constructors of mythic parenting and childhood ideals', *Childhood*, DOI: doi:10.1177/0907568213496657 [Accessed 17/02/2014].

Giddens, A. (1991) *Modernity and Self-Identity: Self and Society in the Late Modern Age*, Cambridge: Polity Press.

Harman, V. & Cappellini, B. (2015) 'Mothers on display: Lunchboxes, social class and moral accountability', *Sociology*, 49(4):764–781.

Hartman, A. & Vining, P. (2007) 'Clinical aspects of the ketogenic diet', *Epilepsia*,

Hays, S. (1996) *The Cultural Contradictions of Motherhood*, New Haven and London: Yale University Press.

Hoffman, D. (2010) 'Risky investments: Parenting and the production of the "resilient child"', *Health, Risk and Society*, 12(4):385–394.

Jackson, S. & Scott, S. (1999) 'Risk anxiety and the social construction of childhood', in D. Lupton [Ed] *Risk and Sociocultural Theory: New Directions and Perspectives*, Cambridge: Cambridge University Press, pp. 86–107.

James, A., Curtis, P. & Ellis, K. (2009) 'Negotiating family, negotiating food: Children as family participants?' in A. James, A. Kjorholt & V. Tingstad [Eds] *Children, Food and Identity in Everyday Life*, Basingstoke: Palgrave Macmillan, pp. 35–51.

Kaplan, E. (2000) 'Using food as a metaphor for care: Middle-school kids talk about family, school, and class relationships', *Journal of Contemporary Ethnography*, 29 (4):474–509.

Lee, E., Bristow, J., Faircloth, C. and Macvarish, J. (2014) *Parenting Culture Studies*, Basingstoke: Palgrave Macmillan.

Lee, E., Macvarish, J. & Bristow, J. (2010) 'Risk, health and parenting culture', *Health, Risk and Society*, 12(4):293–300.

Lupton, D. (1996) *Food, the Body and the Self*, London: Sage.

Lupton, D. (1999) *Risk*, London: Routledge.

McKie, L., Bowlby, S. & Gregory, S. (2004) 'Starting well: Gender, care and health in the family context', *Sociology* 38(3): 593–611.

Metcalfe, A., Dryden, C. & Jackson, M. (2009) 'Fathers, food and family life', in P. Jackson [Ed] *Changing Families, Changing Food*, Basingstoke: Palgrave Macmillan, pp. 93–117.

Meyer, A. (2007) 'The moral rhetoric of childhood', *Childhood*, 14(1): 85–104.

Neal, E.G., Chaffe, H., Schwartz, R.H., Lawson, M.S., Edwards, N., Fitzsimmons, G., Whitney, A. & Cross, J.H. (2008) 'The ketogenic diet for the treatment of childhood epilepsy: A randomised controlled trial', *Lancet Neurology*, 7(6): 500–506.

Payne, N., Cross, J.H., Sander, J.W. & Sisodiya, S.M. (2011) 'The ketogenic and related diets in adolescents and adults', *Epilepsia*, 52(11):1941–1948.

Prior, L. (2003) 'Belief, knowledge and expertise: The emergence of the lay expert in medical sociology', *Sociology of Health and Illness*, 25:41–57.

Shirani, F., Henwood, K. & Coltart, C. (2012) 'Meeting the challenges of intensive parenting culture: Gender, risk management and the moral parent', *Sociology*, 46 (1):25–40.

Vincent, C. & Ball, S. (2007) '"Making up" the middle-class child: Families, activities and class dispositions', *Sociology*, 41(6):1061–1077.

Webster, M. & Gabe, J. (2016) 'Diet and identity: Being a good parent in the face of contradictions presented by the ketogenic diet', *Sociology of Health and Illness*, 38(3):123–136.

Webster, M. (2018) 'Siblings' caring roles in families with a child with epilepsy', *Sociology of Health and Illness*, 40(1):204–217.

Whelan, E. (2007) '"No one agrees except for those of us who have it": Endometriosis patients as an epistemological community', *Sociology of Health and Illness*, 29(7):957–982.

Wheless, J.W. (2008) 'History of the ketogenic diet', *Epilepsia*, 49(8):3–5.

Chapter 13

Concluding remarks

Benedetta Cappellini, Charlotte Faircloth and Vicki Harman

While we were finalising this manuscript, various media outlets reported news of rising levels of obese children worldwide. Reporting new figures from a study based at Imperial College, London, many commented on how childhood obesity had risen from 1975 (when there were 5 million obese girls and 6 million obese boys) to much higher levels today (50 million obese girls and 74 million obese boys) (*The Guardian* 10/10/2017). Discussions of such figures appear periodically in the news, typically accompanied by an analysis of the cost of treating obesity and possible ways of tackling it.

Like other scholars from across the disciplinary spectrum, we find these data alarming and concur that obesity needs to be studied, understood and discussed. However, as social scientists, we also think that a useful step forward in understanding this phenomenon is to reflect on the way it is studied and represented. Looking at how we discuss, research and think about children's diets and well-being can reveal moralising discourses which can arguably prevent rather than help our understanding of this complex phenomena.

In reviewing recent coverage of childhood obesity, for example, we might make the following remark about terminology. Obesity is typically described as an *epidemic*, a medical term referring to infectious diseases, with the implication that obesity is an unstoppable infection. This is not confined to the press, but has become the standard term used by numerous public health agencies, including the World Health Organisation. Academic publications also use this term without distinguishing between its medical and colloquial meaning. Our suggestion, as social scientists, is that the use of such terminology is in itself revealing, enabling a quick slide from a medicalised metaphor into a moralised blame-game. Furthermore, as the papers in this volume show, such accusations of blame seem to be particularly severe for some individuals, couples and groups and less so for others. For example, in the *Telegraph* (10/11/2015) the columnist Julia Hartley-Brewer writes:

> If you are the parent of a fat child, you are a bad parent. Did everyone get that? Because it really is very simple: if your child is overweight then

that is your fault because you are not doing your job as a parent properly. [...] So why do so many parents make their kids fat? Because they are, to put it bluntly, selfish and lazy [...] Demand that the parents come into school to learn how to do the job of parenting properly. And if they refuse, then call in the police and social services and make them do it.

Coverage of recent research studies in the media seems to lend weight to such accusations of poor parenting, informing us that, for example, 'working mothers have fatter children' (the *Daily Mail* 27/06/2016) and that the longer mothers work the fatter their children (The Huffington post 02/04/2011). Such a stigmatisation operated by the media echoes some academic literature adopting a nutritionist perspective, in which parents are described as virtuous when they feed their children with food considered healthy (Horne et al. 2008; Bathgate and Begley 2011) or overindulgent when the food provided is branded and ready-made (Roper and La Niece 2009). Even older generations cannot be trusted to care for children properly, with a swathe of recent stories about 'indulgent grandparents being bad for children's health' (BBC News 15/11/17). These discussions provide an understanding of 'what' type of food parents (or grandparents) provide for their children, but they fail to tackle crucial questions, such as 'how' they make dietary decisions for their children and 'how' children consume food. Focussing discussions only on 'what' food is being consumed and 'what' weight children are, risks providing simplistic, flattened narratives of 'good' and 'bad' parenting without fully unpacking some of the complexities and intimacies of the choices carers face daily in preparing food for children. More broadly, we are suspicious of accounts that seem to demonise certain types of family life, parenting styles and women's lives, not least because research and media operate in an iterative relationship. To put it another way, we have yet to see a study looking at possible links between working fathers and obese children.

Considering the co-constitutive relationship between media and academia, policies and institutions are also influenced by the above mentioned debates. In June 2015, for example, a written question about the powers schools have to inspect children's packed lunches was received in the House of Lords, where Lord Nash responded that schools have common law powers to search pupils and this can be extended to the content of pupils' packed lunches. Lunch box searching has now been established in many schools, with one story about the initiative reporting that 10-year-old pupils are being appointed as 'packed lunch police', inspecting junior students' packed lunches and giving warning slips if food does not meet the school's standards (the *Daily Mail* 28/09/14). The media also reported parents' strong reactions to such initiatives, including protesting against the 'fat letters' that schools sent to parents whose children are considered obese (*The Independent* 10/11/2015).

Such examples point to a complex state of affairs between families and institutions like schools, where the balance of power when it comes to issues such as feeding children is sometimes unclear. But beyond pointing to terminology, what can social scientists and sociologists in particular, offer to this debate? How can sociological work contribute to a better understanding of this complex issue of 'feeding children'?

A first contribution that sociological work can offer, demonstrated in this volume and as noted above, is to move away from simplistic investigations of *what* children eat and *why* they do so, considering instead *how* children eat. Asking questions such as how, why and when, rather than simply what, opens up a richer, if arguably more difficult subject of study, looking at how food is thought of, imagined and desired by children and the adults around them. Exploring how children and adults consume food can facilitate a more nuanced understanding of the everyday practices in which food is included and provide an understanding of how such practices can facilitate or ostracise certain ways of eating and sharing food.

Secondly, looking at how food is/is not available to children at certain food occasions might shine a light on structural aspects dominating dietary choices. As such, investigating how and when certain food is shared can provide a better understanding of the micro and macro aspects affecting children's diets. Looking at the structural aspects of food provision is not a simple task. However, as some pieces included in this volume have shown, 'how' is a question that can best be answered via interdisciplinary research, in which sociological work is paired up with, for example, socio-historical analysis, anthropological perspectives or consumer research studies. An advantage of these interdisciplinary investigations – in which ethnographic work is framed within literature from various disciplinary approaches – is that micro and macro aspects of food and everyday life can be unpacked, looking at how their changes have been affected by the marketplace and how such aspects have been reshaped over time. Furthermore, interdisciplinarity allows for a richness in our theoretical toolkit, drawing on a wide range of concepts – whether that be risk-consciousness, identity work or social solidarity – to push our investigations further.

Finally, sociological work can contribute to a better understanding of the complex issue of feeding children by studying different socio-cultural contexts. Moving away from the dominant Anglo-Saxon perspective of childhood and family life within much of the academic literature provides innovative and more nuanced ways of understanding how the increasingly globalised notions of 'good' parenting, childhood and family life are shaped in different contexts. Also, looking at continuities and discontinuities of such notions across socio-cultural contexts offers a critical understanding of how gendered, racialised and classed structural inequalities affecting family lives and childhood are at play in different ways in various cultural contexts.

To conclude, there is a need for critical sociological work to further unveil structural inequalities and injustices affecting children and their families. Considering the rise of popular views providing simplistic answers to complex questions around family life, we argue that sociological work needs to continue its mission to contextualise the apparently 'objective' language of science and nutrition and to denounce the unplanned effects of some policy interventions. Finally, with regard to food work as well as other areas of family life, it is important to reclaim a more inclusive understanding of what 'good' parenting and 'good' childhood look like: one that works for the many, not only the privileged few.

References

Bathgate, K. and Begley, A. (2011) 'It's very hard to find what to put in the kid's lunch': What Perth parents think about food for school lunch boxes, *Nutrition and Dietetics*, 68(1), 21–26.

BBC News (15/11/2017) Indulgent grandparents "bad for children's health", www.bbc.com/news/health-41981549

The *Daily Mail* (27/06/2016) Working mothers 'have FATTER children': Rise in obesity is blamed on women going out to work, www.dailymail.co.uk/health/article-3662309/Working-mothers-FATTER-children-Rise-obesity-blamed-women-going-work.html

The *Daily Mail* (28/09/14) The packed lunch police aged just 10: They check for unhealthy food in younger pupils' meals – but parents are not happy, www.dailymail.co.uk/news/article-2772966/The-packed-lunch-police-aged-just-10-They-check-unhealthy-food-younger-pupils-meals-parents-not-happy.html

The *Guardian* (10/10/2017) Shocking figures show there are now 124 million obese children worldwide, www.theguardian.com/society/2017/oct/10/shocking-figures-show-there-are-now-124-million-obese-children-worldwide

Horne, P.J. Hardman, C.A. Lowe, C.F., Tapper, K., Le Noury, J. Madden, P., Patel, P. and Doody, M. (2009) Increasing parental provision and children's consumption of lunchbox fruits and vegetables in Ireland: The food dudes intervention, *European Journal of Clinical Nutrition*, 63, 613–618.

The Huffingtonpost (02/04/2011) Childhood obesity: The longer mum works, the more overweight the kids, www.huffingtonpost.com/2011/02/04/childhood-obesity-_n_818385.html

The Independent (10/11/2015) Fat letter sent by school should be scrapped, say experts, www.independent.co.uk/life-style/health-and-families/fat-letter-sent-by-schools-to-parents-should-be-scrapped-say-experts-a6728891.html

The Telegraph (10/11/2015) If your child is fat then you are a bad parent, www.telegraph.co.uk/news/health/11985974/If-your-child-is-fat-then-you-are-a-bad-parent.html

Roper, S. and La Niece, C. (2009) 'The importance of brands in the lunch-box choices of low-income British school children', *Journal of Consumer Behaviour*, 8(2–3), 84–99.

Index

acculturation 29
adaptation of behavior by children 134
advertising 145
aesthetics of food 56–9
agency 109
Aitken, S. 153
Alaimo, K. 90
Allison, A. 30
Andersen, Sidse S. 44
"Anglo-Saxon" perspective on childhood and family life 157, 209
Anving, T. 117–18, 126
Asian families 18
authoritarian approach to eating in school 44

babies, feeding of 4
Bach, D. 12
Ball, S. 192
Banwell, C. 193
Beck, U. 192
Beck-Gernsheim, E. 192
"becoming" concept (*becoming-the-same* and *becoming-other*) 125, 130–5
Blair, Tony 45
Blumberg, S. 98, 101
Bolivia 5, 63–81
Boltanski, Luc 43–7
Brakes (company) 91–3
"breadwinner" role 144, 152–3, 157, 160, 169
breakfast brought from home 19–21
breakfast eaten at home 170
breakfast schemes 91
Brembeck, H. 127
Burman, E. 11
Butler, P. 96

calibration of motherhood 174–7, 180, 186–8
Cappellini, B. (co-editor) 193, 200
care work *see* childcare
Cascais 48–51, 54–5, 59
Centros de Desarrollo Infantil (CDIs) 69–70, 77–9; meetings at 74
Centros Infantiles (CIs) 68–9, 77–80; food shopping for 71–3; meetings at 74; school fees for 73
child centres (in Bolivia) 63–70, 76–81
child rearing: expert advice and guidance about and supervision of 2; importance, complexity and expectations of 2
child-centeredness 3, 158
childcare responsibilities 149, 153, 156–8, 169–70, 193, 198, 203
Children North East 92
Children in Scotland 92
children's role, change in 121
Chowbey, P. 30
"civilising" of children 12–15, 18–19, 24–5
convention theory 44–7, 51, 60
Cook, J. 89
Cook, Robin 28
cook–chill meals 51–4
cooking 156–70, 175; children involved in and taught about 167, 181–2; as a hardship 162, 164–6; as an interest 162; men's ability at 166–9; as part of life 162, 167–8; philosophy of and attitudes to 164–5, 168–9; by women 193
Coskuner-Balli, G. 160, 168
Coveney, J. 79
Crenshaw, Kimberlé 28

Crowley, R.H. 13–14
Crozier, G. 66, 79
Cuff, M.E. 13–14
culinary femininities and masculinities 158–9, 162, 169
cultural dominance 30
"cultural swapping" 29
Curtis, P. 15, 20, 119–20
custody of children 160

Daniel, Paul 44
De Certeau, Michel 110, 121
Defeyter, M.A. 89
demonisation 208
Denmark 6, 30, 143–4, 148–9, 153–4
deprivation: in childhood 99–100; measurement of 87
Desmond, Matthew 108, 120
desserts, eating of 118–19
DeVault, Marjorie 107, 109, 175
dieting 197; see also ketogenic diet
"Dirty Dozen" list 183
disciplinary power 65–7, 74
divorce 157, 162
Dixon, J. 193
Donner, H. 30
Douglas, Mary 115
Draper, M.C. 64
"dual emancipation" 156–9, 168

early childhood settings 11–19; variation between 23–5
eating, children's: research and policy initiatives concerned with 42; social processes related to 42
eating habits 13, 16–17, 89, 181
eating out 131
eating process 107–21; either *forcing* or *encouraging* children to engage in 117–19; seen as both *conceptual* and *physical* practice 108
"eating scripts" 126, 129, 132
Ecuador 67
Ekström, K.M. 126
Electronic Ketogenic Manager (EKM) 198
Elias, N. 14, 17
Ellis, K. 119–20
emotional labour 198–9, 202–3
epilepsy, treatment for 6–7, 191, 199
Epp, A.M. 152
ethnicity 29, 38–9

ethnographic research 16, 209; relational approaches to 108, 120–1
European Fruit Distribution Regime 50
expert carers 200–4

family identity 135, 152, 158
family meals 6, 12, 15, 79–80, 91, 113, 115, 125–35, 150–1; and identity practice 132–3; pressures on 127–8; as social practice 125–6
family relationships 5, 110, 144
fast food 178
fathers, roles of 4, 6, 143–54, 156–70
Fathi, M. 29
favourite dishes 131
"feeding ordering" concept 43, 54, 59
feeding process 107–21
femininity see culinary femininities and masculinities
feminism 29, 175–7, 183
Field, Frank 92
fish dishes 50–1, 54–9
Fitzpatrick, M. 2–3
Fjellström, C. 159
food: cultural meanings of 44; education about 44, 66, 80, 91; as fuel 163, 169; safety of 52–3
Food Cardiff 91–3
food choices 23, 39, 114–15, 125, 131–4, 151, 175–7, 181, 209
"food events" 12–13, 16, 19, 24–5
"food ideal" 126, 130, 134
food insecurity 87–90, 93–8, 101; effect on health and behavioural problems 89–90; impact in North America 97
food parcels 92
food poverty 5–6
food scarcity 119
foodbanks 90
Foucault, Michel 65–6
free school meals 87–92, 96, 98
fruits, intake and knowledge of 50
Furedi, F. 2
"fussy" mothers 12, 22

gender equality and gendered roles 144–5, 156–9, 198; see also women: responsibilities mainly taken by
gendered nature of food work 197–9
Gill, O. 88
Gilliam, L. 13–14

Gillies, V. 11, 21
Goffman, E. 176
Goldschmeid, E. 15
Good Housekeeping (magazine) 144
Gottzén, L. 159
Gulløv, E. 13–14
Gustafsson, Ulla 44

Hamilton, W.L. 101
Harman, V. (co-editor) 193, 200
Hartlepool Borough Council 92
Hartley-Brewer, Julia 207–8
Hays, S. 3, 192
health, holistic view of 43
health education 181
healthy eating 31, 150–4, 167, 181
healthy foods 44, 75, 79, 128, 175–6, 183, 208
healthy living 2–3
Hochschild, A. 160
Hoffman, D. 192
holiday clubs 6, 87–102; availability of 95, 98, 101; differences in offerings between 101; location of 99–102; rise of 90–2
holiday hunger 87–101; definition and measurement of 95–8, 101; questions for quantification of 97–8, 101; schemes for dealing with 90–3
home backgrounds of children 17–19
hooks, bell 29
hospital admissions 199
Household Food Insecurity Access Scale 97
housework 144–5, 148–53, 158–60
housing standards for children's families and for educators 23
how (as distinct from *what*) food is eaten 208–9

identity *see* family identity; mothering identity; professional identities
Income Deprivation Affecting Children Index (ICACI) 99
individualisation 192
inequalities affecting childhood and family life 209–10
infant experience 2–3
intensive mothering 158, 202–3
intensive parenting 3–7, 113, 192, 195–7, 202, 204; necessity of 195–7
interdisciplinarity 5, 59

intersectionality 28–9, 39
interviews with whole families 148

Jackson, P. 145
Jackson, S. 15
James, A. 15, 119–20, 124, 126
Japan 30–1
Johansson, B. 125, 131, 134
junk food 6, 44, 178–81

Karrebæk, S.M. 30
Kellogg's (company) 91–3
ketogenic diet 6–7, 191–204; positive views of 199–200
Koch, J. 80

Lahire, B. 107–8
Law, John 43–7, 60–1
lay expertise 200, 203–4
Lazar, S. 80
Leahy, D. 66, 79
Lee, E. 2
"lines of flight" 125, 131–5
lunch boxes 11, 21–4, 28–39, 193, 200; case studies of 32–7
Lupton, D. 67, 163

"McDonald's Mom" image 174, 177–83, 186–8
McDonald's restaurants 185–6
MacKendrick, N. 182
Make Lunch (charity) 91
malnutrition *see* nutrition
marginalisation 12
marketing of food 125
Marshall, D. 144–5, 152–3
masculinity 152, 157–64, 167–70
maternal foodwork 175–7, 180, 183, 186–8; standards set for 187
maternal leave *see* parental leave
The Mayor's Fund for London 92
Meah, A. 145
meals (hot) brought from home 21–2
mealtime practices 12, 17
medical monitoring of children 76–8
Mediterranean Diet 50, 55
Medium Chain Triglyceride (MCT) diet 191, 201
mental health 89–90
Metcalfe, A. 37

middle-class backgrounds 21–5, 31, 134, 157–8, 177–8, 187, 192
migrant families 28–9
"militancy" regarding food 183–4
Modified Atkins Diet (MAD) 191
monitoring of food consumption 197
Morales Ayma, Evo 65
moralising 3, 20, 78, 207
Moser, Caroline 67–8
mothering *see* intensive mothering
mothering identity 201, 203–4
mothers 3–4; "good" and "bad" 175–7, 210; overbearing and obsessive 174–5, 182; as perceived by child centre staff 74–5, 81; reported behaviour at child centres 75–6; stigmatisation of 174
multiculturalism 28–9
Murcott, A. 79–80

Nash, Lord 208
neoliberal policies 64–5, 100–2, 188
Neuman, N. 159
Northeast Childhood Poverty Commission 96
nutrition 93, 163, 195; awareness of 75–81

obesity in children 44, 49, 59, 64, 77–81, 188, 207
Ochs, E. 125–6
Office for Standards in Education (OFSTED) 20
Oliver, Jamie 45–6
"orders of worth" 45–7, 60
"Organic Child" ideal 176
"Organic Mom" image 6, 174, 177–8, 182–8
Ortner, S. 109
Osgood, J. 19
outsourcing 51
Owen, J. 145, 152–3

packed lunches 21–2, 30, 150, 179–80, 208; *see also* lunch boxes
parental leave 149, 153, 157
parenting: and children's food consumption 196; culture of 1–4; goal of 29; new type of 144, 170; standards of 22, 31, 38, 66, 79, 176, 207–10; styles of 6; *see also* intensive parenting
parents, non-biological 145
parents' eating 113

parents' meetings 74, 79
partnership between educators and children's families 12, 25, 66, 81
paternal leave *see* parental leave
Piagetian perspectives 124
Pike, J. 66, 79
Pinstrup-Andersen, P. 97
planning of meals 193, 195
Portugal 5, 42–60; school meals reform in 49–51, 59–60
poverty 87–8, 96–102; as regards both money and time 67; stigmatisation of 98–9
Price, L.L. 152
Pristavec, T. 182
private sector provision of services 24–5, 100–1
private sphere 80
problematic children 22
professional identities of educators 24
professional identities of some parents 21, 24, 160–1, 168–70
Promotion of Healthy Eating (PNPAS) initiative 50
public policy 11, 102
public provision of services 24–5

racism 187
ready-made meals 169
resistance: to family meals 128, 132; to school meals 44, 51, 54–9
restaurants, use of 196
"risk society" concept 192
Romani, S. 128

Scandinavian context 153
school holidays 5–6
school kitchens, establishment or refurbishment of 51–4
school meals 5, 42–60; biomedical understanding of 43; children's resistance to 44, 51, 54–9; reform program in Portugal 49–51, 59–60
school meals supervisors 14
school powers 208
school regulations 30–1
Schroeder, K. 65
Sellerberg, A.M. 117–18, 126
separation of child from mother 22
Sharma, N. 88
Shinwell, J. 89
Shoher, M. 125–6

shopping 150–2, 195–6
single fathers 156–8; *see also* fathers, roles of
snacks 129–30, 133–4
social class 29–30, 39, 152, 188
social isolation 98–9
social judgement 186
social problems 88
social relationships and interactions 121
social rules 116
social skills 88, 101
social support 94
socialisation 14, 124–35, 181, 188; in reverse 125–6, 135
societal norms 204
socio-cultural contexts 209
sociological work 209–10
stigmatisation 98–9, 102, 168, 174–82, 187–8, 208
strategies, parental 110, 115–21
Strathern, M. 108–9
StreetGames (charity) 92
stress 89–90
structural adjustment policies 64–7, 81
summer learning loss 89
surveillance 1, 5, 63–7, 78, 174, 188
Sustain organisation 92
Sweden 6, 156–9, 168
Szabo, M. 158, 169

table manners 13–14, 17–18, 116
tactics, children's 110, 119–21
takeaway meals 131–3

Tanner, C. 145–8, 152–3
targeted support 95
tastes in food: demarcation and synchronisation of 126–7; development of 120, 126–7
"tasting evenings" 23
teacher-trained educators 24
Thévenot, Laurent 43–7
Thompson, C.J. 160, 168
time, allocation of 67
"top-down" development 78
Townsend, Nicholas 143
"treats" for children 176, 185
Truninger, Monica 43
Trussell Trust 90

Vertovec, S. 28
vignettes 148
Vincent, C. 31, 192
vulnerability of children 4, 124–5

Webster, M. 191–2
Weinreb, L. 89
Welch, R. 79
women: employment of 80–1, 149, 157, 178, 208; responsibilities mainly taken by 109, 152, 156–8, 175, 193, 198–9, 202–3
working-class backgrounds 14, 19, 25, 31, 66, 177, 187 192
World Bank 65
World Food Summit (2006) 97
World Health Organisation 207

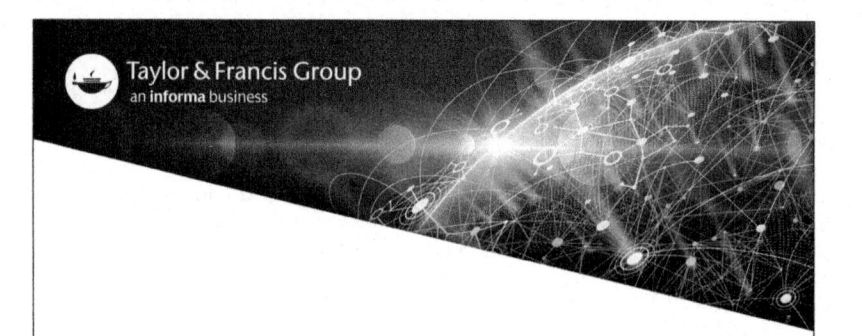